COMFORT COOKING

for Bariatric Post-Ops
and Everyone Else!

Lisa Sharon Belkin

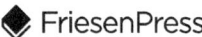 FriesenPress

Suite 300 - 990 Fort St
Victoria, BC, V8V 3K2
Canada

www.friesenpress.com

Copyright © 2018 by LISA SHARON BELKIN
First Edition — 2018

All rights reserved.

The author's reference to various brand-name products are for informational purposes only, and are not intended to suggest endorsement or sponsorship by the author or her book to any company or owner of any brand. The author advises the reader to take precautions in using recipes where known food allergies may be of concern. The author disclaims any liability personal or otherwise resulting from the use and information in this book.

No part of this publication may be reproduced in any form, or by any means, electronic or mechanical, including photocopying, recording, or any information browsing, storage, or retrieval system, without permission in writing from FriesenPress.

Front cover photograph: Salisbury Steak (page 84 with Faux Mashed "Potatoes" page 120)
Back cover: Cheesecake (page 184), Cobb Salad (page 62), Chicken Pot Pie (page 98), Tomato Soup (page 60)

All photographs, food styling and designs by Lisa Sharon Belkin.

ISBN
978-1-5255-2281-9 (Hardcover)
978-1-5255-2282-6 (Paperback)
978-1-5255-2283-3 (eBook)

1. COOKING, HEALTH & HEALING, WEIGHT CONTROL

Distributed to the trade by The Ingram Book Company

DEDICATION

For all of us who continue to climb
the stairs to success, I dedicate this book.
May you find joy and comfort on your journey
—Bon Appétit!

ABOUT THIS BOOK

I HAVE ALWAYS ENJOYED COOKING AND BAKING. AS AN ARTIST, I HAVE EXPRESSED MY CREATIVE JUICES in the studio. Out of necessity, I decided to develop and create masterpieces in my kitchen as well. What a wonderful merger! For the past year I have focused my creativity as a recipe developer to bring you the most delicious comforting foods that make us feel warm and tingly inside and at the same time are "pouch worthy" for us bariatric post-ops. Bariatric surgery is more common place now than it was fifteen years ago but even now there are still very few cookbooks out there that can help us on our journey. Yes, there are low-carb, low-fat, diabetic, high-protein, and a host of other books available, however the recipes are not specifically designed for people who have had bariatric surgery (we require protein rich, pouch worthy, soft, tender, juicy and saucy) or have a history of sugar and food addiction. I am not a doctor or a nutritionist. I have been gifted a tool to work with in my weight loss journey and have since lived a bariatric lifestyle. This book includes a master grocery list for everything you will need to have in your fridge, freezer, and pantry to make the recipes in the book as well as tips and ideas for preparing and freezing portions so that you will never have to make another impulsive drive thru run or make other bad food choices because you were pressed for time or there was nothing in the house. These recipes have helped me lose 175 pounds over the course of six years post-Lap-Band surgery. I hope that they become a part of your journey to success and I wish you the same enjoyment that they have given me. Best of luck to you all!

Lisa Sharon Belkin

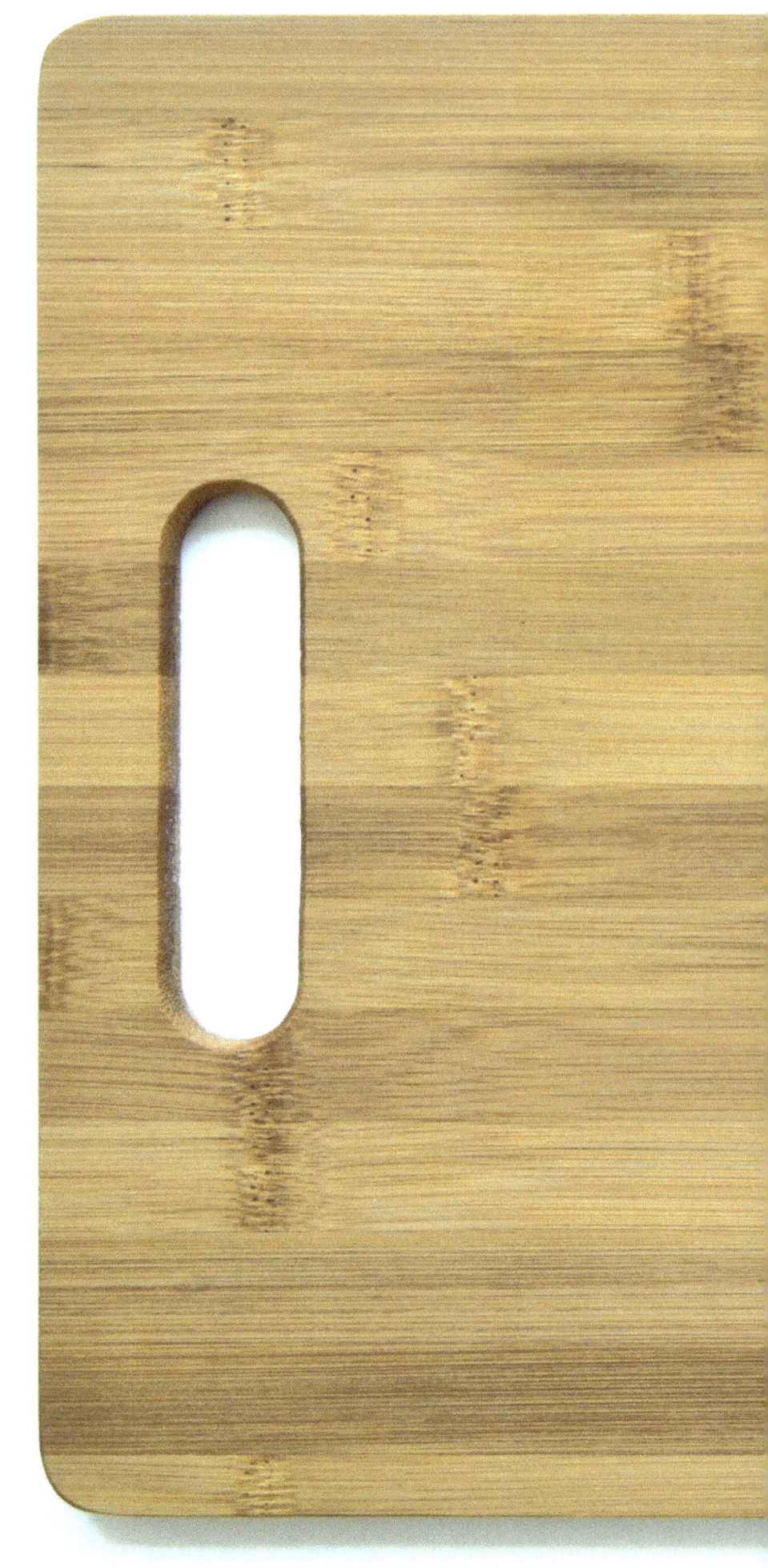

TABLE OF CONTENTS

About This Book v

Introduction ix

A Few Words About.................. xiv

Protein Snack Ideas and Tips............ xix

Concluding Remarks xx

The Recipes..................... 1

Appetizers 3

Beverages..................... 37

Soups And Salads.................. 49

Main Dishes.................... 71

Sides And Vegetables................ 117

Gravy And Sauces 149

Desserts 161

References..................... 204

My Bff 204

About The Author.................. 206

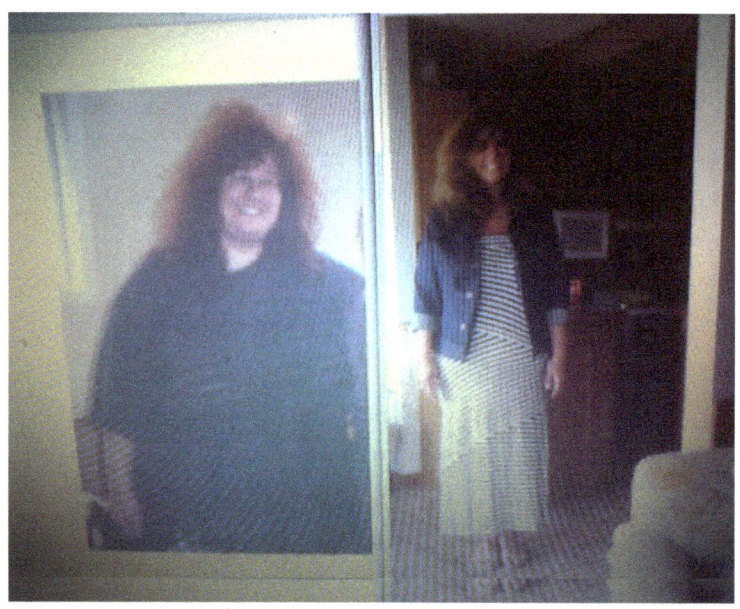

Bless the girl on the left and continue to bless the girl on the right who worked hard and continues to work hard each and every day.

INTRODUCTION

Fail to prepare, prepare to fail —Benjamin Franklin

WHILE DOING RESEARCH FOR THIS BOOK, I CAME ACROSS A BRUTALLY HONEST AND WONDERFULLY insightful personal explanation of the weight-loss journey that has become my "mantra" and, I believe, will become yours too. There was no reference to any name as to who said it. All I know is that it struck a familiar chord with me. Read it slowly and carefully every day for the next few weeks until it really sinks in and becomes a part of who you are. It will change your attitude about commitment and, inevitably, it will help you to reach your goal. A woman who lost half her weight was asked how, how fast, and what she had to give up to lose the weight. This is what she said:

1. It has taken me every day. Not six weeks, not six months. Every day. I start again every day.
2. I gave up bad habits one at a time. I gave up excuses. I gave up blame. I gave up sugar and bad carbs. I gave up short cuts and fake stuff.
3. I took advice from my body about what was working and what wasn't. I took advice from people who had won, not people still at war. I focused on one path instead of chasing miracles.
4. I celebrated every win. Some days it was a new number or a new size. Some days it was an airplane aisle without turning sideways. Some days it was someone saying, "All the cute clothes are for little people like you." Some days it was just being able to put the bread down, spit the sugar out, or stop before regret! And honestly, some days I celebrated being able to start again tomorrow.
5. I made time for success. I prepped, I planned, I scheduled it. Success in anything has to be scheduled.
6. I quit waiting for a better time.

So there you have it. Beautiful, almost poetic, and a great answer for all of us if we are asked the same question. Believe in it and learn it well so that it falls from your lips automatically.

***

After nearly six years of receiving the gift of a gastric band (with a few bumps along the way), I finally figured out the key to success in my weight-loss journey. As most people know, bariatric surgery is just a tool, and, after the first few years, it becomes much harder to lose and stave off regain. I have the answer. I stumbled on it accidentally. While we can and should continue to follow our surgeon's recommendations and plans, this book will give you additional help by offering you simple, delicious, and satisfying meal options that are high protein, low in carbohydrates, and sugar free, which you can mix and match. The recipes are divided into categories that will help you organize your meal planning. I am not a doctor or a nutritionist; I can only give you my personal experience as a post-bariatric patient, living in the real world, who is working hard to get to my goal and not battle the regain with which many struggle. Ultimately, your bariatric team should be consulted about any issues that you may be having. I just want to offer you my wonderful recipes that have helped me stay on track. I do recommend, however, that you make sure you take your daily vitamin requirements, drink your water, have a daily whey protein isolate drink or two (this staves off hunger in between meals and helps us attain our daily protein requirement with very few calories and carbs), and get enough sleep and exercise. Also, have your blood work done regularly and meet with your bariatric doctor as scheduled. These are all a part of healthful living and nothing new. But in your hands, you now hold a wonderful book that will be an extra tool for you to help meet your goals. Enjoy the ride and start cooking!

Out With the Old, In With the New

It is no secret that I am a food addict. If you are a post-bariatric patient, then you and I are the same. We love food, period. We didn't grow to be 300-plus pounds eating salads and grapefruit. We didn't have our intestines rerouted, 85 percent of a healthy organ cut out or a plastic implant placed to almost choke out our stomachs just because. We had it done because after years of countless diets and regimes that we've all tried, only to fail and gain it all back, we had one last option that offered us hope. We chose surgery and it IS a difficult path. So after it is all said and done, here we are. At some point after the "honeymoon stage" (one or more years out from surgery), we are left to wonder what and how to eat to continue to lose weight or maintain the weight we have lost without gaining any of it back. Some of us already have seen dreaded regain and now wonder if we will ever be able to eat the same foods and treats (albeit in smaller portions) that we ate pre-surgery. The answer is simple. No. In the olden days, diets meant fruit, vegetables, lean meats, very little fat, and usually two pieces of bread daily, etc. and little else. No wonder it was hard to stick to a plan. At that time, surgery was not an option, and we only heard of it on rare occasion. We had only one thing that we could rely on to help us stick to our diets and it was called WILL-POWER. Well, I never quite found my will-power. Even to this day. I realized that there is no will-power and I am too old to look for it. Looking back to my dieting history before surgery, conjuring up the will-power was always torture. Having to refrain from eating things I wanted was truly horrible. You know what I'm talking about. We have all relied on our will-power. Ahem . . . well, my will-power, or lack of, got me up to almost 400 pounds. The only answer for me was surgery and that helped me get down to a more normal weight. To date, I have lost a total of 175 pounds and counting. However, it is not as easy now as it was the first few years. I have concluded that your surgeon is responsible for your weight loss for the first few years but, after that, it's all in your hands. I came to know this as I approached year three and four after surgery and found that, somehow, I was starting to make bad food choices and nibbled on things from which I should have stayed clear. Namely, the same things that grew me to almost 400 pounds; of course, the amounts were much smaller, however the frequency was becoming alarming to me. Something drastic had to be done because I saw into the future and could see that, if I continued on this path, I would end up gaining back all or most of the weight that I lost. Surgery was a help, but it was not going to stop me from making bad choices. I really thought the surgery was the last stop for me to finally end my quest for thinness, but reality hit hard as I pondered the inevitable. Light bulb moment here. And this is where the phrase *necessity is the mother of invention* took hold of me. I became obsessed with the idea of how to turn this thing around. And as it started to take shape, I realized that the best part was that I did not have to rely on will-power anymore. I just had to resolve to prepare everything I loved in a new way and completely ditch the things that made and kept me fat. Of course, I still had to make the right choices and do the preparations, but it was easier this time. Because the food was so good, I did not feel like I was missing out on anything. Best of all, the scale is moving again in the right direction. I can honestly say that I love to cook again! I lost my passion for cooking in the first few years after being banded, but I got it back! Okay, so now let's talk about food.

As a post-bariatric patient, we all know that we must give up sugar. Recently, it has become known that the sugar industry has been putting our lives at risk since the early 1960s. A recent *New York Times* article stated that internal historical documents from the Sugar Association were accidentally discovered by a researcher at the University of California at San Francisco and it revealed over five decades of research showing the link between sugar and heart disease. In the *New England Journal of Medicine*, where the reviews of the sugar research were published, the findings were minimized by paying off Harvard scientists to play down the results in an effort to conceal the truth and instead promote saturated fats as the leading culprit in heart disease.[1] Sugar has also been linked to whole-body inflammation. In his bestselling book *Wheat Belly*, William Davis, MD, presents many examples that illustrate how inflammation in the body is intensified in the presence of high blood sugar levels after ingesting sugar and wheat. The long-term damage of sugar wreaks havoc in the body and is responsible for many serious ailments. One such quote from the book is as follows:

> So high blood sugars that encourage growth of a wheat belly, coupled with inflammatory activity in visceral fat cells and glycation of cartilage, lead to destruction of bone and cartilage tissues in joints. Over years, it results in the familiar pain and swelling of the hips, knees, and hands.[2]

This I found most interesting because I personally suffered from sore muscles for years. I had difficulty walking up and down the stairs, and getting up from a chair or couch, because of pain and stiffness. I attributed it to getting old. Interestingly enough, after eliminating sugar and bad carbs from my eating, within three weeks, I caught myself going up and down the stairs with ease, and realized that the pain and soreness in my body had disappeared. It was, indeed, miraculous. And I knew that the link between sugar, bad carbohydrates, and my body pain were all related. We all kind of know that sugar is bad for us, but I don't think that we quite know how bad. For food addicts, sugar is like crack. Once in the blood stream, the effects of sugar bring on a euphoria that feels so darn good, only to be followed by crashes that bring on intense cravings for, you guessed it—MORE sugar. This never-ending, roller-coaster of sugar and cravings is what made us fat to begin with. We cannot stop eating. Sugar makes us SUPER-HUNGRY! It's very hard to ask will-power to step in when you become a hungry ogre who needs a fix of sweets, or potatoes, bread, pasta, crackers, chips, etc. (yes, all of these convert to sugar), and so on and on it goes.

Now, continuing to build my case, here is another revelation for you! Remember in all your past attempts at losing weight when you were told by your doctor or dietitian to eat everything in moderation and you will be fine? (Early on for me was when I was eight years old—yes, I have been on this journey of weight loss since I was a kid.) Well . . . now, for some bariatric post-ops who have learned the hard way, the big buzz statement in the bariatric world is "Everything in moderation is a big fat lie."

The theory with this is that, in the first few years after surgery, you could practically eat whatever you wanted, you could even deviate from your surgeon's guidelines and somehow still lose weight. Wait a minute!!?? How is this possible? Well . . . as you know, the first twenty-four months post-op is often called the honeymoon phase. Basically your surgeon is responsible for your weight loss. This means that after the surgery, your body is adjusting to the new wiring of your insides and your pouch is still healing and you are quite diligent to not overeat. You lose weight even if you have a bite of this or that. For these couple of years, you are not in the driver's seat. But what happens after the honeymoon phase is over is entirely up to you. You are now driving the bus and suddenly you find your weight loss is stalling or, worse yet, REGAIN happens. After eating everything in moderation for a few years, suddenly the scales start moving up, up, up, and even though you still are not eating the way you did pre-surgery, the dreaded regain happens. Why? Because eating sugar and bad carbs makes us hungry. It's logical to say then that if you go with the "everything in moderation" theory, and you eat bread and a little piece of cake, or that fast-food burger and small fries, it will all convert to sugar and you won't be able to stop! Some of you have been going down this path, and I am sure you get it. I saw myself going down this path and I could see that history would repeat itself even AFTER bariatric surgery! We were never able to moderate those foods before surgery, and most of us are unable to moderate those foods after surgery. You wouldn't suggest to a crack addict to "just have a little" would you? Reality check, people. This is us—except our drug is sugar and bad carbs.

So there you have it, and here is where I will explain about this cookbook. I love food but I cannot and will not jeopardize my hard work only to ingest things that will get me off track, and make me gain weight and go through a detox session again. That means starting again "tomorrow"—especially after having a love affair with chocolate and potato chips for months. You all know how hard it is to get back on the wagon. It's painful. So let's not torture ourselves anymore and let's not rely on will-power. I assure you that if you adopt these recipes and this new way of eating into your daily life you won't want to touch anything in the pantry that you shouldn't. But let me add: it's always easier to clean up your environment if you can. This means: get rid of trigger foods in your house if you can. Actually, if you think that you can't because your kids love potato chips and jelly beans, or your husband loves taco chips at night while watching television, think about how much you love them all

and look for alternatives that are healthier for them as well. It is important to mention here that all the recipes in this book are family-friendly and will pass the taste test of even the most skeptical, finicky eater! There is no need to prepare meals for you AND different meals for your family! WIN-WIN!

But what can I eat, you may ask? The key is to learn to make your favourite foods but tweak them so that they don't contain any refined sugars or nasty carbohydrates. This whole new way of preparing food has brought back the joy and creativity to cooking that I have missed for many years. In the last few years, I have become a recipe developer and my kitchen has become a test kitchen for my wonderful recipes. I've revamped my old scrumptious comfort food recipes and replaced them with practically identical ones with no compromise to flavour or texture. I have also developed new recipes, and they have now become staples in my bariatric life. I urge you to start incorporating some of the recipes in this book into your daily life. Remember, the idea is to eliminate sugars and bad carbs from your food choices and replace them with healthier versions. Do this, and you will stay in control and on track. Once you get the hang of things, you can start to tweak some of your own family favourites that you abandoned since surgery, and add them to your repertoire. Some recipes, however, may not be able to be tweaked. Don't worry; the recipes here may be the only ones you want or need.

This book is all about comfort with food that is healthy, delicious, and easy to prepare. It has been said that food should be looked at as fuel for our bodies and nothing else. We are not cars. I have to be honest with myself. Food is more than fuel to me. We humans are not like animals. We have used food for more than nutrition. It has become our entertainment and our pleasures. Food means fun, friends, and family. And even as bariatric post-ops, food still has to bring pleasure to us and, at the same time, meet our nutritional requirements, too. How can we stay on a good program of eating, with some familiar comfort foods, without putting us at risk of gaining weight? This book includes a collection of over ninety revamped recipes of my favourite things that you can prepare for breakfasts, lunches, and dinners. There is even a section for special-occasion desserts. I have also included a list of over fifteen easy, high-protein snack ideas.

The recipes are quite simple, ever-so-tasty, bariatric-friendly and will become your BIBLE. I make these recipes in rotation and never get tired of them. Feel free to tweak them with more or less spice if you choose.

If you take a survey of most households, you will find that people tend to buy the same things over and over and tend to eat the same things again and again in rotation. This is the same idea. Having so many wonderful choices will help you with daily or weekly menu planning. Both ways will keep you on track and loving every bite.

You don't have to deprive yourself of anything. You just need to learn how to make your favourite foods bariatric-friendly and so tasty that you won't need to ever deviate from them. This book will be your new normal. You just need to believe in yourself, and change the way you prepare your food. You will have that light bulb moment too, and it will become effortless.

The recipe categories include appetizers, beverages, soups and salads, main dishes, sides and vegetables, gravy and sauces, and desserts. A few words about desserts. Desserts (cakes, pies, and cookies) are not something we should be eating after every meal. These treats are for special occasions like birthdays, anniversaries, and holidays, so that we can also participate at the end of the meal without sabotaging our efforts. They are so good that you could serve them to anyone. So if you are entertaining or have a party to go to, don't convince yourself that you won't be tempted by the sweet treat on the table or the dessert offered at the end of the meal. Make or bring something that you can enjoy too and you won't fall off track. Everyone loves a good cheesecake! For me, I enjoy an occasional afternoon cup of decaf coffee and I usually enjoy it with one (see that?), one, of my homemade cookies that sit in a jar on my kitchen counter. In the past, a jar of cookies would never last a week on the counter. However, today, one cookie is enough because without the load of sugar, there is no need or no desire for another. One satisfies without guilt or compulsion to eat the entire jar. It is so bizarre. If you told me that I could leave a jar of cookies on the kitchen counter and only have one with a cup of coffee and it would be enough, I would have never believed it. With my past track record, this concept was completely inconceivable. Also, the longer the cookies stay in the jar, the crunchier they become and I look forward to a really good, crunchy cookie now and then! Having this ritual helps me stay on track.

The key to using this cookbook with the most effective outcome is to find the recipes you enjoy the most in each category and make them over and over again in rotation. This will not be hard. To me, they are all winners. Embrace them.

A FEW WORDS ABOUT

Breakfast

MOST POST-OPS ARE NOT VERY HUNGRY IN THE MORNINGS BUT IT'S STILL IMPORTANT TO FUEL YOUR body within one hour upon arising. This is a great time for a protein shake. I use a whey protein isolate. Not a protein blend. Be sure to read your labels well. Whey protein isolate is the purest form of protein and the body can absorb most of it. Protein blends have a mix of proteins and the body does not absorb very much of it. Be creative with your shakes. I usually buy the chocolate and the vanilla, but, when I use the vanilla, I usually add pumpkin spice or sugar-free flavoured syrups like Starbucks or Torani. You can also add peanut butter powder to the chocolate shake or a flavoured extract. I always make my shakes with unsweetened almond milk. If shakes are not your thing, have a Mini Quiche (page 34) instead. One more thing about protein shakes. In order to meet your daily protein requirements, you would have to eat a serious amount of meat, dairy, etc. Protein shakes can get you to your daily protein goals for very little calories and carbs. If you cannot tolerate a protein shake in the morning, have one for a snack sometime during the day or evening. I understand it's difficult for many to drink a cold drink in the morning. Here's a good trick. Sometimes I will add a scoop of my protein powder to my coffee mug, mix it with a few tablespoons of room temperature water until it's smooth, then add my coffee (you have to slowly temper it into the protein otherwise you will get a globby mess). This is a delicious way to have your coffee in the morning with a good dose of protein to get your morning started. Again, if you use a protein blend, this might not work. It may be too gritty. You need a protein isolate that will mix up smoothly in liquid.

Sugar

For all sugar replacement needs I use Truvia Baking Blend, Truvia Brown Sugar Blend, and Stevia In The Raw granular form. Truvia Baking Blends combine Truvia calorie-free sweetener (stevia leaf extract), erythritol, and a tiny amount of sugar (yes, a tiny amount of sugar, however, we are talking about having an occasional portioned dessert that will not trigger cravings for more or make you super-hungry), which results in an overall product that maintains the sugar-like taste and texture but with 75 percent fewer calories from sugar. Truvia Baking Blends do contain calories and carbohydrates, so make sure that you account for them in your eating plan. I do not have regular sugar of any kind in my home. That includes honey. For me, Truvia blends work very well for my baking needs and yields a better result than other granulated sweeteners. Whether I am baking cakes, pies, or cookies, they always come out perfectly. There is absolutely no strange aftertaste or bitterness. Truvia is twice as sweet as regular sugar, so you would only use half as much. For those of you who still want to continue to use Splenda or any other granular sweetener, that's fine. The desserts in this book use Truvia Baking Blend, so if you choose to use any other granular sweetener, remember to double the amount. Again, I will mention that for baking, Truvia blends are my preferred choice.

Personally, I would rather eat and serve a really good piece of whatever, than compromise taste and texture by using other granular sweeteners. It is your choice. You have options. Remember that the recipes in the dessert section, other than the protein chews and the crunchy protein cinnamon cereal, are designed for special occasions and holidays. Enjoy an occasional guiltless treat with everyone else!

Flour and Bread Crumbs

There are times when you just cannot avoid white flour. Therefore, some of the recipes call for white flour or Bisquick baking mix. You will notice that the amounts are VERY scaled down and are usually combined with almond flour and/or parmesan cheese. You are never to eat an entire recipe, only one portion at a time. The amount of carbs in a portion of each recipe is very minimal and should not trigger cravings. You should be satisfied with a single serving. The same goes for dry bread crumbs and panko. Again, there is such a small amount being used in the entire recipe, so there should be no worries about consuming one serving. I have found that you can cut down on these two ingredients quite a bit and use them sparingly, however, you cannot eliminate them completely.

Portions

If you have had obesity surgery, your pouch (restriction) should determine your portions. I don't list portions because of this. We are all different, but generally our pouches decide when it's enough and we need to be aware of the cues when we've had enough. For some, it is a hiccup, for others a sneeze. The cues vary but I am sure you know which one belongs to you. If you feel you are eating more than you think you should and are banded, I suggest you talk to your surgeon, as you may need an adjustment. If you adapt these recipes into your eating plan, you shouldn't be feeling ravenous when you sit down to a meal; therefore, a small portion should be enough. If you eat your protein first, then vegetables, etc. there should be no issues with overeating. As we have a built-in portion control mechanism, if we choose the proper foods, measuring becomes an option. Also, remember to never drink with your meals, eat slowly, use small plates and utensils, chew each bite twenty times and wait thirty seconds between bites. If you can't seem to wait the thirty seconds, sit on your hands—this should help.

Portioning and Freezing

I do this A LOT! My freezer has so many of my favourites already portioned out, so it's incredibly convenient to just decide what I want, pop it on a plate, and microwave it. This is especially wonderful on days that I don't feel like cooking or have no time to cook. One of my all-time favourite things is my Chili (page 74). I usually make a huge pot of it and then divide it up and freeze it. It is always on hand. I love to bake, and I often have a variety of cookies frozen as well. When you cook any of the recipes and have leftovers, freeze them into portions. Sometimes, when I have extra time, I will prepare a casserole, like the Lazy Perogy Casserole (page 138), cut it into nine equal portions and freeze them individually. I often make a double recipe of Italian Meatballs (page 80) and freeze them in large freezer bags. Do this enough times with different recipes and you will always have something delicious that can be on the table in less than twenty minutes. I also like to buy rotisserie chickens, de-bone them, discard the skin then chop up the meat and portion it out to freeze so I can put together a Comfort Chicken Bowl (page 100) any time. Keeping your freezer bariatric-friendly and stocked with single servings is an excellent way to stay on track every time!

Grocery List

You were born to win, but to be a winner you must plan to win, prepare to win and expect to win.
—Zig Ziglar

This is really a must. I have created a master grocery list, with all the things you need to make every recipe in this book. This will make grocery shopping very easy. Print out a few copies and keep one close to you. It will help you to become super-organized, and guarantee that you have everything you need. Your fridge, pantry, and freezer will never again leave you without options, which we all know can lead to making poor choices. The items on the list are all basically low in carbohydrates, and will, therefore, yield only low-carb meals. Here is the list of foods and items organized by category that you should have in your house at all times. This list excludes other items that your family, household, and pets may require.

Master Grocery List

Meats and Seafood

- Deli meats (lean turkey/ham and no-sugar-added types)
- Bacon and breakfast sausage
- Italian sausage
- Chicken breast/thighs (skinless/boneless)
- Ground chicken/turkey*
- Rotisserie chicken
- Salmon/other fish fillets
- Extra lean ground beef (chuck)
- Prepared lean burgers for grilling*
- Shrimp (raw)/scallops* /crab (not imitation)
- Beef hot dogs (fat-free or close)*
- Roast (chuck)
- Ribs
- Pork tenderloin*
- Pepperoni slices

Cheese

- Laughing Cow light wedges
- Fat-free cheese slices
- Mozzarella cheese (reduced fat)
- Ricotta cheese (reduced fat)
- Cottage cheese (1%)
- Cheddar cheese (reduced fat)
- Babybel Gouda (light)
- Cream cheese (reduced fat)
- Parmesan cheese
- Blue cheese

Eggs/Milk/Dairy/Non-Dairy

- Eggs
- Unsalted and salted butter
- Unsweetened almond milk
- Sugar-free Cool Whip
- Whipping cream
- Plain Greek yogurt (0%)
- Sour cream (low fat, <u>not</u> fat-free)
- Milk (skim, 1% or 2%)
- No sugar, low-fat coffee whitener (International Delight)
- Soft margarine (Becel)

Vegetables and Fruit

Red and green peppers	Celery/carrots
Fresh ginger	Bean sprouts
Cauliflower	Garlic
Avocado	Sweet potato (white flesh)
Zucchini	Coleslaw mix
Jalapeno peppers	Frozen spinach, chopped
Onions	Romaine/iceberg lettuce
Cucumbers	Spaghetti squash
Brussel sprouts	Frozen mixed vegetables
Mushrooms	Tomatoes
Cabbage	Lemons/limes
Green onions	Granny Smith apples
Broccoli	Fresh and frozen strawberries, blueberries, raspberries
Green beans	(no sugar added)

Cans/Jars/Bottles

No aroma coconut oil	Peanut butter (low sugar)
Sesame seed oil	Peanut butter powder
Extra virgin olive oil	Sugar-free preserves, all flavours (Smucker's)
Ketchup (Heinz, no sugar added)	Apple sauce (no sugar added)*
Yellow and Dijon mustard	Maple syrup (no sugar added)
Beans (kidney, black, pinto, chick peas, refried, etc.)	Soy sauce
Hellmann's mayonnaise, half fat	Tuna/salmon (canned)
Salsa (no sugar added)	Caesar salad dressing, half fat
Tomato sauce (no sugar added)	Alfredo sauce
Tomato paste	Flavoured extracts (vanilla, almond, etc.)
Bolthouse yogurt salad dressings	Regular and decaf coffee granules
Sriracha sauce	Vegetable cooking spray
Hot sauce (tabasco, Frank's)	Liquid smoke
Pumpkin puree (not filling)	Canned soups (low sugar and no pasta or rice)*
Green beans, canned	White vinegar
Diced tomatoes, canned	Worcestershire sauce
Pickles/olives/artichoke hearts	Water chestnuts

Packaged Items

Stevia, raw granular sugar substitute	Chocolate, vanilla, and unflavoured whey isolate protein powder
Truvia Baking Blend	
Truvia Brown Sugar Blend	Almonds/walnuts/pecans/pistachios
Unsweetened cocoa powder	Panko bread crumbs
Skim milk powder	Dry bread crumbs

COMFORT COOKING
for Bariatric Post-Ops and Everyone Else!

Low-sodium chicken and beef stock
Beef/chicken bouillon packets (Oxo, Knorr)
Bisquick baking mix
Baking powder/baking soda/cream of tartar
Almond flour **AND** white flour
Pork Rinds*
Beef/turkey jerky
Cornstarch
Sugar-free, semi-sweet chocolate chips
Sugar-free cookies (oatmeal, shortbread)
Quaker instant oatmeal flakes
Sugar-free chocolate/vanilla/butterscotch pudding mix

Sugar-free Jell-O, varieties
Sugar-free candies (Werther's, Sweet'N Low)*
Sugar-free popsicles and Fudgsicles*
No-sugar-added ice cream (watch carbs and sugar alcohols)*
Quest protein bars
Bagged, fully cooked bacon flakes*
Small bag raisins/unsweetened dried cranberries
Turkey/chicken/mushroom gravy mix
Foil/plastic wrap/Ziploc lunch and large freezer bags, parchment paper, wax paper

Spices

Oregano
Poultry seasoning
Rosemary
Thyme
Chili powder
Cumin powder
Curry powder
Seasoning salt
Black pepper
Sea salt
Paprika
Garlic powder
Ground cloves
Ground nutmeg

Cinnamon
Cayenne pepper
Dried Italian blend
Dried onion flakes
Dried parsley
Ground ginger
Pumpkin spice
Old bay seasoning
Dried dill
Onion powder
Red pepper flakes
Popcorn seasoning shakers, all flavours
Ranch dressing powder
Onion soup mix*

Beverages, etc.

Lemon/lime concentrate
Diet cranberry cocktail, Ocean Spray 10
Torani/Da Vinci sugar-free syrups
Flavoured water enhancers, all flavours
Sugar-free lemonade powder mix (Crystal Light)
Smooth Move Tea*
Ice*

* Extras (not required for any recipe but good to have on hand)

LISA SHARON BELKIN

PROTEIN SNACK IDEAS AND TIPS

- Zero percent plain Greek yogurt with a few squirts of flavoured water enhancer or berries
- Babybel/Laughing Cow light cheese with ten green grapes
- One-quarter cup almonds with cheese
- Movie goodie bag (almonds, Babybel cheese, grapes)
- Scoop of protein powder mixed into zero percent plain Greek yogurt. As an option, use vanilla protein powder in yogurt, warm for fifteen seconds in the microwave then drizzle with sugar-free maple syrup and top with one tablespoon chopped walnuts and a few crunchy protein cinnamon cereal pieces (see Desserts) for a warm, comforting bowl of mock cereal.
- Cottage cheese with sliced cherry tomatoes
- Hardboiled/devilled eggs/olives or dill pickle slices
- Whey protein isolate shake
- Apple slices/Laughing Cow light
- Beef/turkey jerky (low or no sugar added)
- Few slices deli turkey or ham rolled with mustard and low-fat cheese
- Protein bar (watch the sugar and carbs; I recommend Quest bars as they are low-carb, high fibre and one gram of sugar per bar and have 21 grams of protein.)
- Any of my soups with an added scoop of unflavoured whey protein isolate (one that mixes smoothly in liquid)
- Protein Chews (see Desserts)
- One-half cup Crunchy Protein Cinnamon Cereal (see Desserts)
- Hummus/guacamole (see Appetizers) with cucumber slices
- Sugar-free Jell-O with a dollop of plain Greek yogurt sweetened with any granular sweetener or a squirt of any flavoured water enhancer

Tip One: Sometimes you just need a sweet in your mouth. I have a few sugar-free candies and this usually does the trick. Stock up on them when they are on sale. I love them in all flavours. Be aware of the sugar alcohols, though, as they are not completely absorbed in the digestive system and therefore cause bloating or abdominal discomfort in some people. For me, I don't notice any reaction and so I have a sugar-free candy now and again.

Tip Two: It's a good idea to have a snack with you on hand just in case. There will be times when you are running late and will not make it home in time for your meal and you will be hungry. Have portable protein snacks in your office drawer, purse, or car at all times. Almonds, jerky, protein bars, and a few single servings of protein powder that mix well with water are some examples. Never be caught off guard. Not being prepared opens the door to bad choices.

CONCLUDING REMARKS

Spread Your Wings and Fly

I HOPE THAT I HAVE INSPIRED YOU TO EMBRACE YOUR KITCHEN AND MAKE WONDERFUL BARIATRIC-friendly comfort foods. Prep work is the key to success and making sure you have everything on hand is extremely important. Never leave anything to chance, and make sure you always have a plan in place. Good luck, friends, and remember that everything in life that is worth fighting for is never easy. A book like this will be an additional help for you. Enjoy these recipes and the pleasures they will bring to your life.

> There is no elevator to success. You have to take the stairs.
> —Zig Ziglar

Ending this book with one of my favourite quotes by the American motivational speaker Zig Ziglar seems appropriate. They are words to live by and should be an everyday reminder that there is no easy way to reach our goals, but with the effort, we can get there! Good luck to you on your quest for success!

THE RECIPES

Every recipe has been optimally tweaked with the precise ratio of ingredients needed to obtain the best texture and taste.

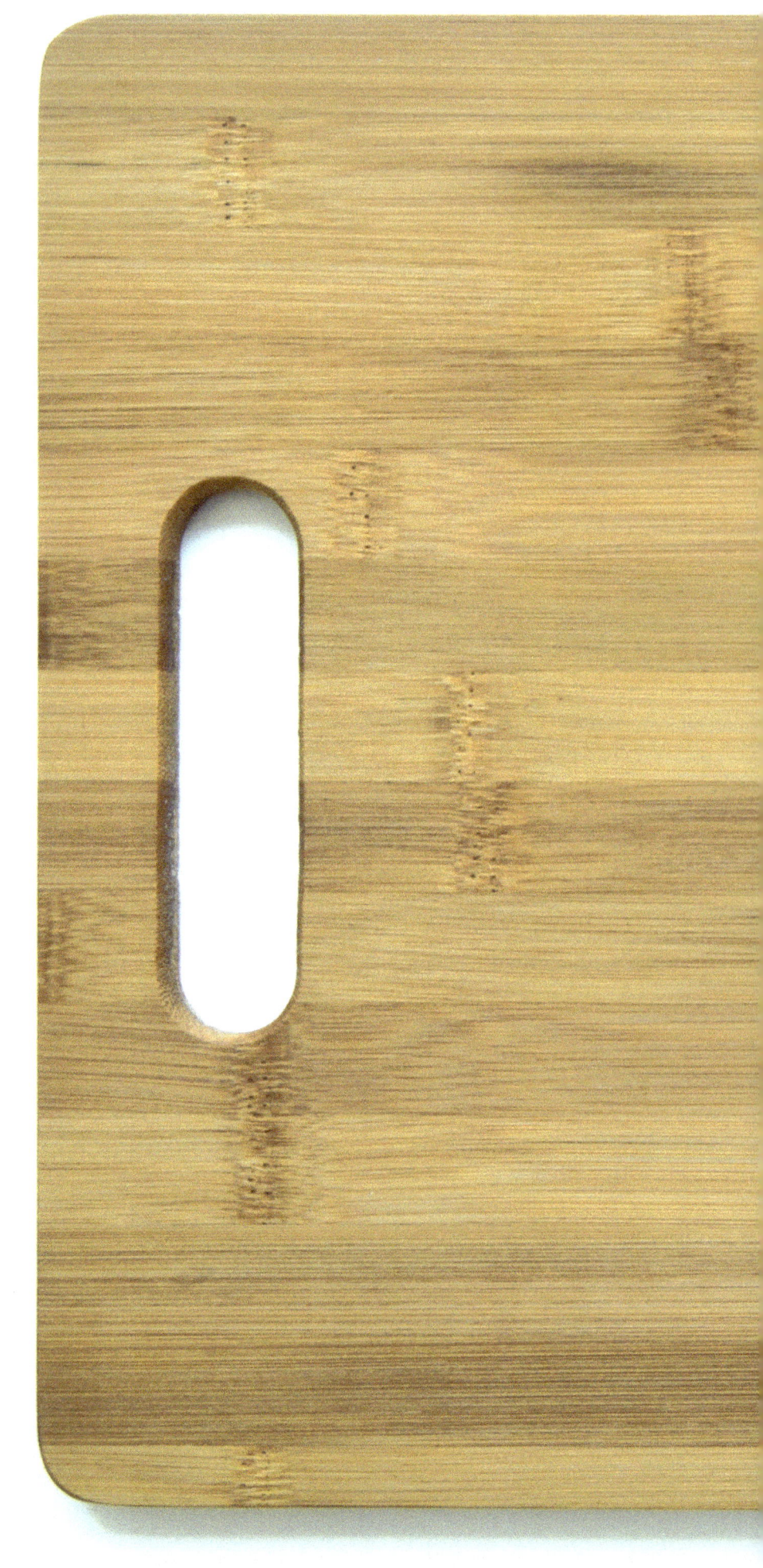

APPETIZERS

Sweet and Spicy Almonds or Pecans 4

Cheese Crackers 6

Cheesy Protein Croutons...................8

Blue Cheese Dip 10

Spinach Dip..............................12

Baked Artichoke and Parmesan Dip 14

Crab Cakes...............................16

Italian Chicken and Zucchini Poppers 18

Buffalo Wing Chicken Balls................20

Teriyaki Wings on a Skewer................22

Hummus...................................24

Yummy Guacamole..........................26

Curried Devilled Eggs....................28

Stuffed Mushrooms 30

Cheese and Chives Brownies 32

Mini Quiches 34

COMFORT COOKING
for Bariatric Post-Ops and Everyone Else!

SWEET AND SPICY ALMONDS OR PECANS

These are a great make-ahead snack to have for a healthy munch (about one-quarter cup serving) or to put out for guests in a lovely bowl on a table of appetizers. Sweet and spicy without a bad carb in sight.

INGREDIENTS

1 t. butter

2½ c. of almonds or pecans (toasted)

1 T. water

1 T. Truvia Brown Sugar Blend

1 t. olive oil

2 T. sugar-free maple syrup

¼ c. Truvia Baking Blend

1 t. cayenne pepper

1½ t. coarse salt

INSTRUCTIONS

1. Melt butter in a large skillet and toast nuts over medium heat. Stir constantly to avoid burning and just until oils are released and almonds are slightly browned, about five minutes. Remove from heat.

2. In a small bowl, blend water, Truvia Brown Sugar Blend, olive oil, and sugar-free syrup until well mixed. Add to the nuts and toss to coat. Return to low heat and continue to coat until liquid has evaporated and nuts are dry to the touch. Transfer to a cookie sheet and spread in a single layer. Cool slightly.

3. Place Truvia Baking Blend, cayenne and salt into a large plastic freezer bag. Seal and shake to mix, then add the almonds. Seal and shake to coat. Place the almonds back to the cookie sheet, spreading in a single layer. Let air-dry for several hours. Store in an airtight container.

NOTE: For a real treat, you can add one teaspoon of cheesy caramel corn popcorn seasoning into the freezer bag with the other ingredients. I use Kernel Season's brand, which has zero grams of carbs and zero grams of sugars per serving.

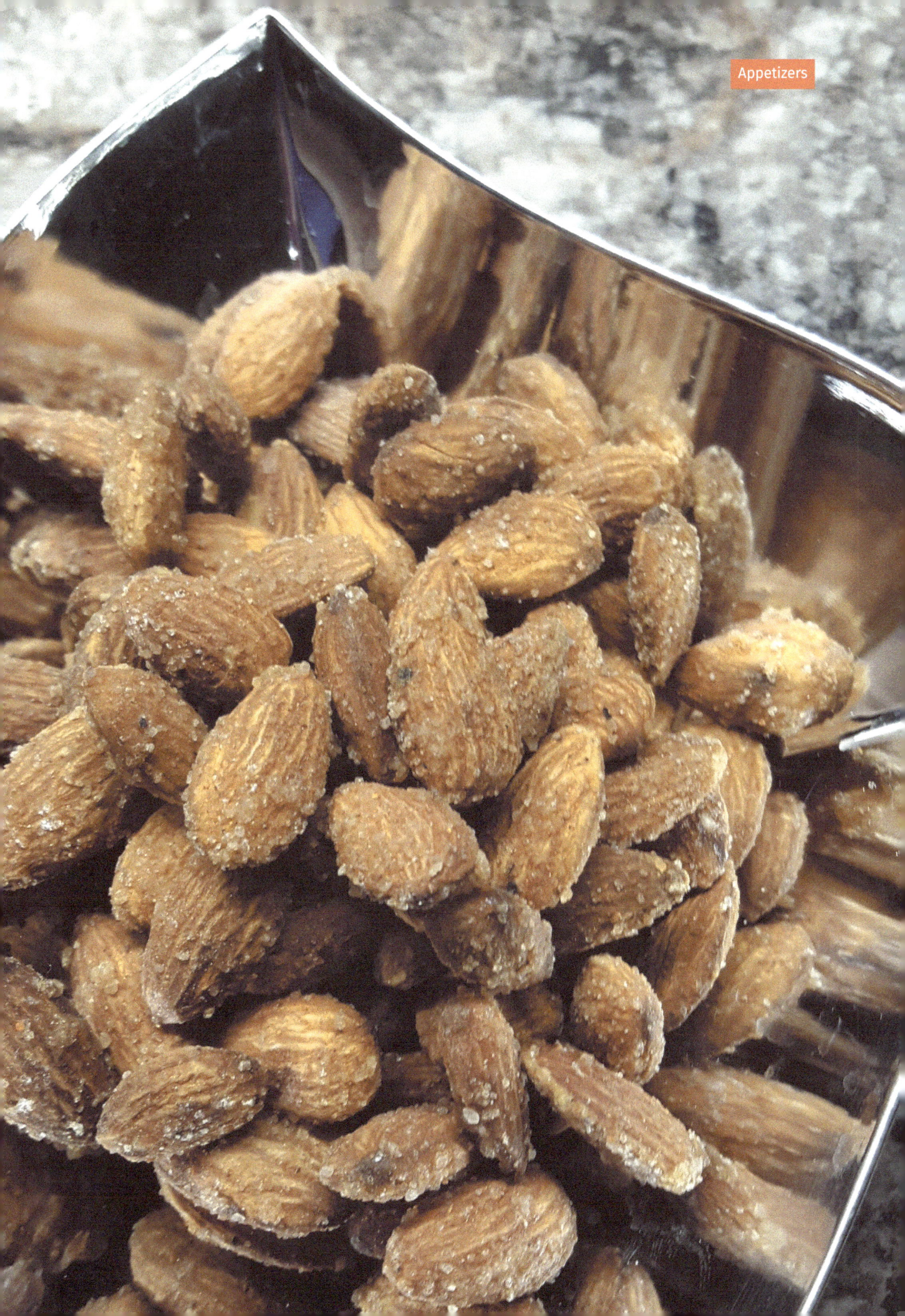

Appetizers

COMFORT COOKING
for Bariatric Post-Ops and Everyone Else!

CHEESE CRACKERS

These crackers are the bomb. They can be made plain or you can sprinkle them with any popcorn flavouring powder to suit your mood. A beautiful addition to a cheese tray, cut up vegetables, and dips.

INGREDIENTS

- ¾ c. almond flour
- ¼ c. white flour
- ½ c. reduced-fat cheddar cheese, shredded
- 1 egg white
- ½ t. garlic powder
- ¼ t. black pepper
- 1 t. onion powder
- ¼ t. salt
- 1 T. dried parsley
- ¼ t. cayenne pepper (optional)

INSTRUCTIONS

Pre-heat oven to 275°F.

1. In a medium-sized bowl, combine ingredients and mix well. With clean hands, form a dough ball and set down on a large rectangular sheet of parchment paper.

2. Place a sheet of parchment paper on the dough ball and roll the dough into a rectangular form, as thin as you can. Remove the top parchment paper and transfer the rolled dough onto a cookie sheet. Cut away any overhanging paper to clean things up.

3. Using a knife, score the dough into long strips about two inches wide and then score in the opposite direction so you will be left with squares. You can score each square diagonally to form triangles. This is entirely up to you. Get creative!

4. Bake for 30 minutes, making sure they do not burn. If you like them a bit darker then by all means bake them a little longer. Remove from oven and let cool slightly.

5. Break the long strips first, then break apart each square, and, if you scored each square into triangles, break each square. Leave the crackers on the cookie sheet in a single layer and let them cool completely till they crisp up.

6. Sprinkle the crackers with any popcorn flavouring or leave plain. Store in an airtight container.

NOTE: An easier alternative is to form dough into one log, cover with plastic wrap and freeze for one hour. Slice thinly and bake as directed. Don't forget to line the baking sheet with parchment paper.

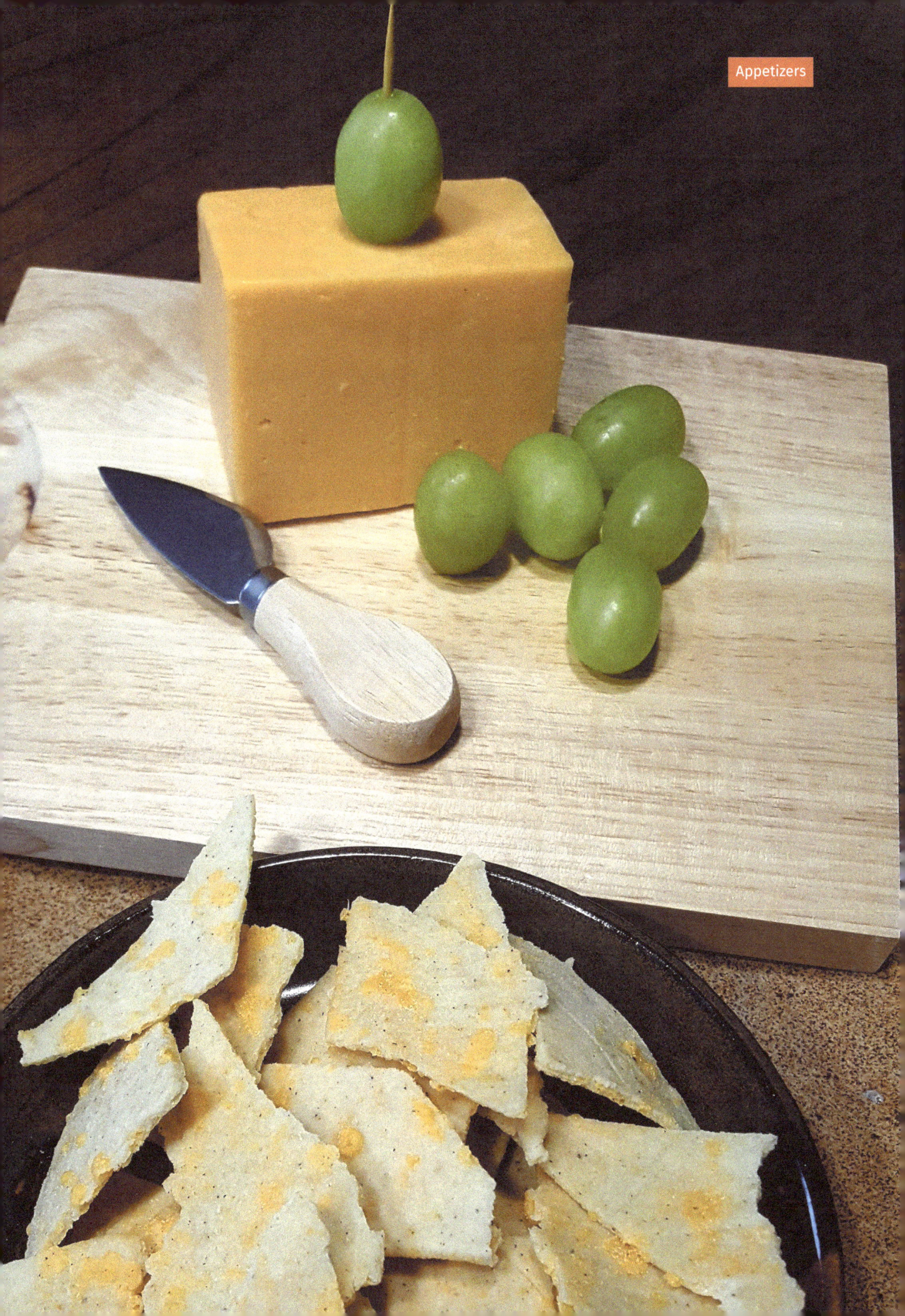

Appetizers

CHEESY PROTEIN CROUTONS

Add a few of these to top off your soup or salad. You can also enjoy these with a hardboiled egg or a few slices of deli meat as a wonderful snack.

INGREDIENTS

¾ c. almond flour

¼ c. white flour

1 scoop unflavoured whey protein isolate powder

1 egg white

1 t. garlic powder

¼ t. onion powder

½ t. salt

¼ t. baking powder

½ c. reduced-fat cheddar cheese, shredded

2 t. olive oil

INSTRUCTIONS

Pre-heat oven to 275°F.

1. Combine all ingredients in a small bowl and mix well to form a dough ball.
2. Take small pieces of dough and roll between your palms into cigar-shaped ropes. You should have about seven or eight ropes.
3. Slice each rope into thin pieces and arrange on a cookie sheet prepared with parchment paper.
4. Bake for 30 minutes or more. Turn them over after 20 minutes and continue to bake for an additional 10 minutes. Be careful not to burn them.
5. Remove from the oven and leave them on the cookie sheet to crisp up and cool. The longer they air-dry, the crispier they will become.
6. Transfer the croutons to a large Ziploc bag and add one-half teaspoon of cheddar popcorn seasoning, one teaspoon parmesan cheese, plus one-half teaspoon garlic powder. Seal the bag and shake to distribute. Store in an airtight container or Ziploc bag.

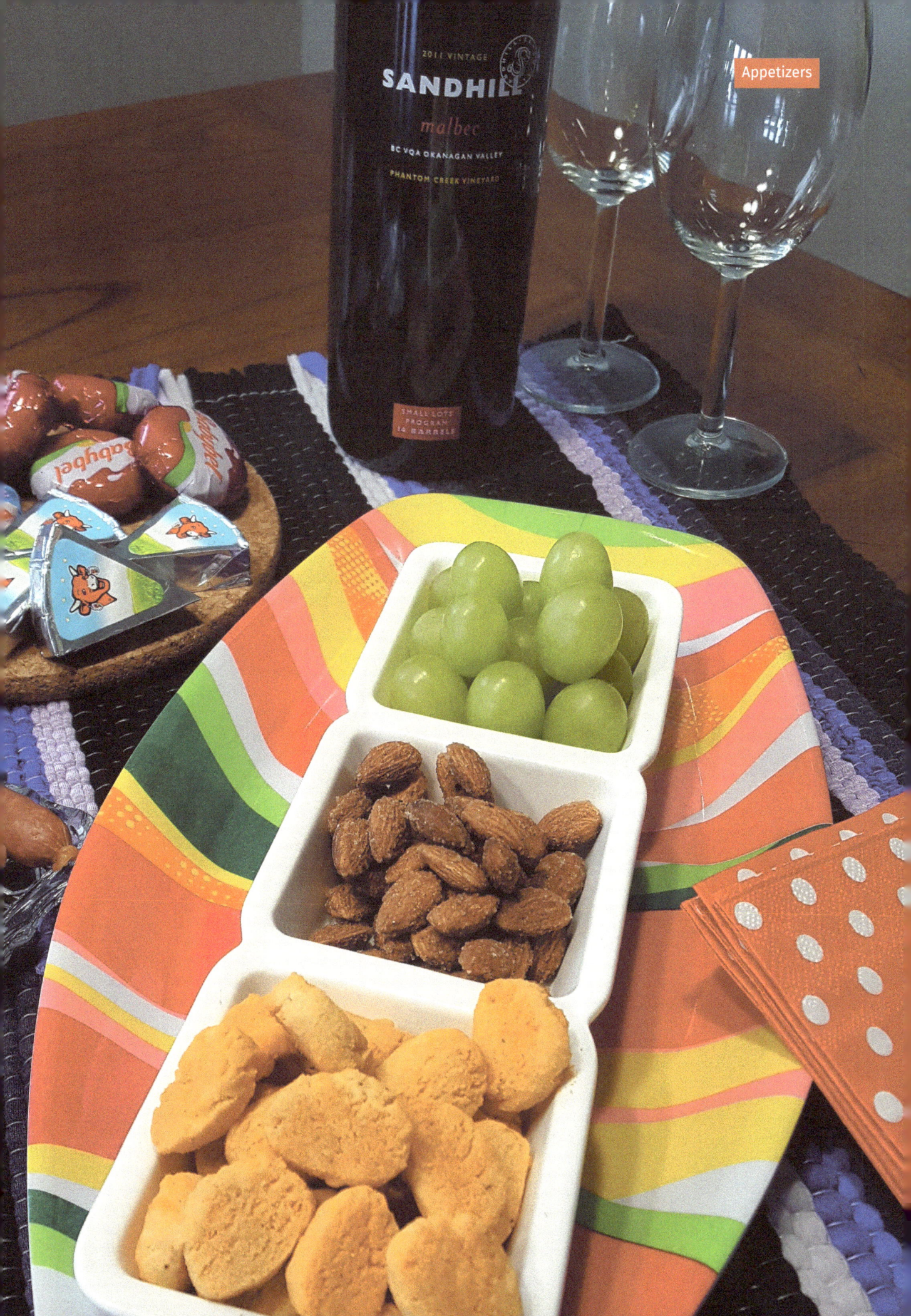
Appetizers

BLUE CHEESE DIP

I love blue cheese anything and this dip will be a hit with everyone. The caramelized onions kick up the flavour to a gourmet level.

INGREDIENTS

1 c. green onions, thinly sliced

1 t. vegetable oil

2 T. half-fat mayonnaise (I use Hellman's)

1 c. 0% or 1% plain Greek yogurt

4 oz. blue cheese, room temperature and crumbled

2 green onions, thinly sliced, plus 2 T. chopped walnuts for garnish

INSTRUCTIONS

1. In a small non-stick pan, sauté the onions in oil over medium heat till nicely browned, about 10 to 12 minutes. At the same time, add a pinch of salt and pepper. Set aside to cool.

2. In a separate bowl, whisk together mayonnaise, yogurt, and blue cheese until well combined and smooth. Stir in caramelized onions and mix well. Season to taste with additional salt and pepper if needed.

3. Spoon into a small bowl or serving dish and garnish with sliced green onions and walnuts.

4. Serve with cucumber chips, red pepper strips, and jicama matchsticks.

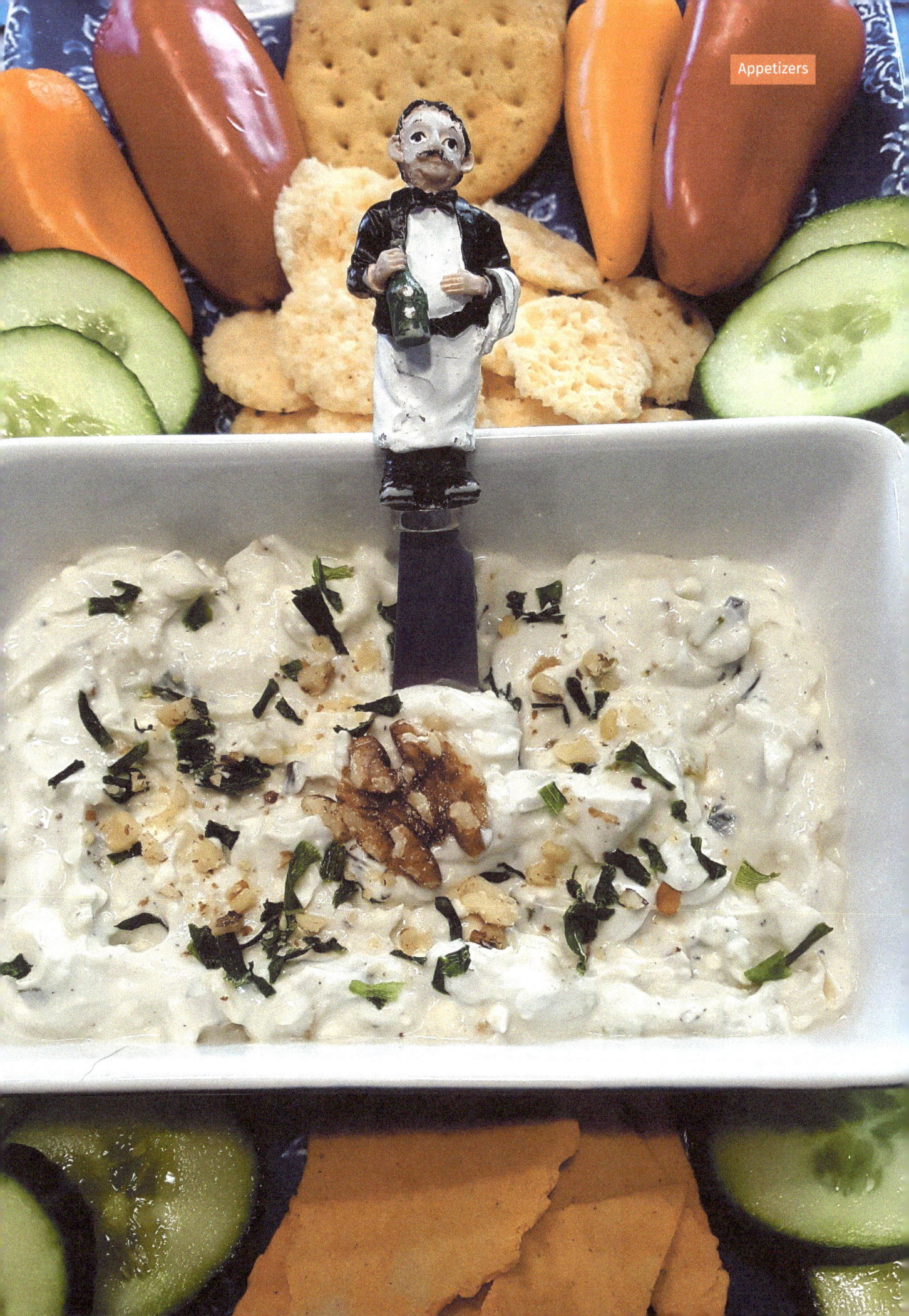

Appetizers

SPINACH DIP

I have always loved spinach dip. This one is just as tasty and you don't miss that pumpernickel bread because you have options. Dip with my cheese crackers and veggie sticks, or even better, just a spoon!

INGREDIENTS

- 2 T. olive oil
- 10 oz. bag frozen chopped spinach (thawed and squeezed dry)
- 1 clove garlic, minced
- 1½ c. 0% plain Greek yogurt
- 1 T. half-fat mayonnaise (I use Hellman's)
- ½ can water chestnuts, chopped
- 1 T. vegetable soup mix (I use Knorr)
- 1 T. green onions, sliced thinly
- ½ t. onion powder
- ½ to 1 t. salt
- ¼ t. pepper

INSTRUCTIONS

1. In a bowl, combine oil, spinach, garlic, yogurt, mayonnaise, water chestnuts, soup mix, sliced green onions, onion powder, salt, and pepper. Taste and adjust salt and pepper if necessary.
2. Mix well, cover, and chill several hours before serving.
3. Serve with a variety of veggie sticks, such as red and yellow peppers, jicama, cucumber slices, apple slices, Wisps, or the cheese crackers found in this book. You can even have a small scoop of it with a few slices of rolled up deli meat as a nice lunch.

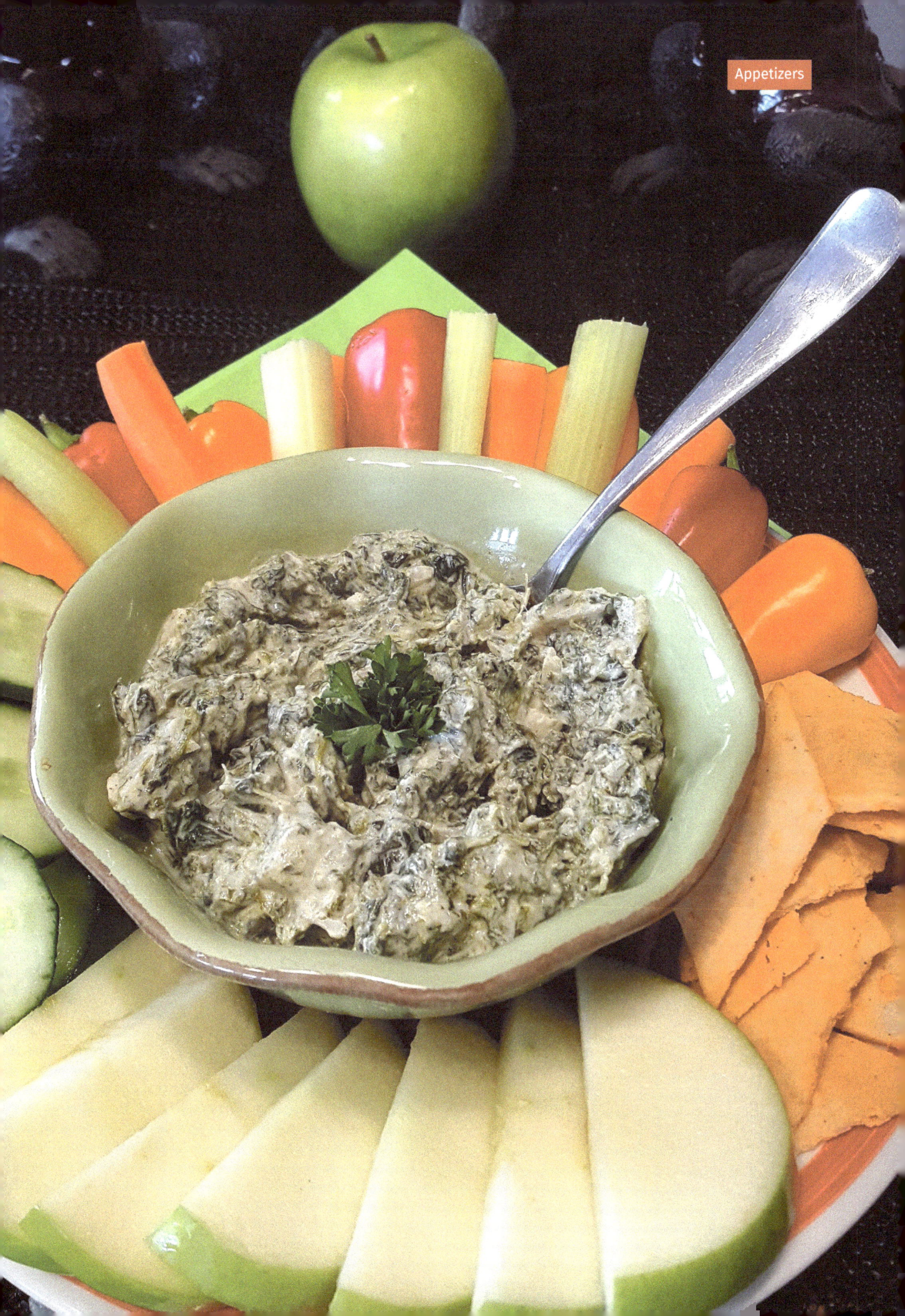

COMFORT COOKING
for Bariatric Post-Ops and Everyone Else!

BAKED ARTICHOKE AND PARMESAN DIP

So, so good. This wonderful dip is a regular item on many restaurant menus but this one has been modified by cutting down the fat without compromising the taste or texture!

INGREDIENTS

One 28 oz. jar, artichoke hearts packed in water, drained and chopped

½ c. parmesan cheese

1 packet of Leek soup mix (I use Knorr)

½ t. garlic powder or 1 mashed garlic clove

1 T. lemon juice

3 T. half-fat mayonnaise (I use Hellman's)

⅔ c. 0% plain Greek yogurt

¼ c. reduced fat mozzarella cheese, shredded

Fresh ground pepper

INSTRUCTIONS

1. In a medium-sized bowl, blend all ingredients till well combined. Spoon into a shallow baking dish and refrigerate until ready to bake.

2. Bake at 375°F for 30 to 40 minutes until browned and bubbly. Serve with crackers, pita crisps, apple slices, and celery.

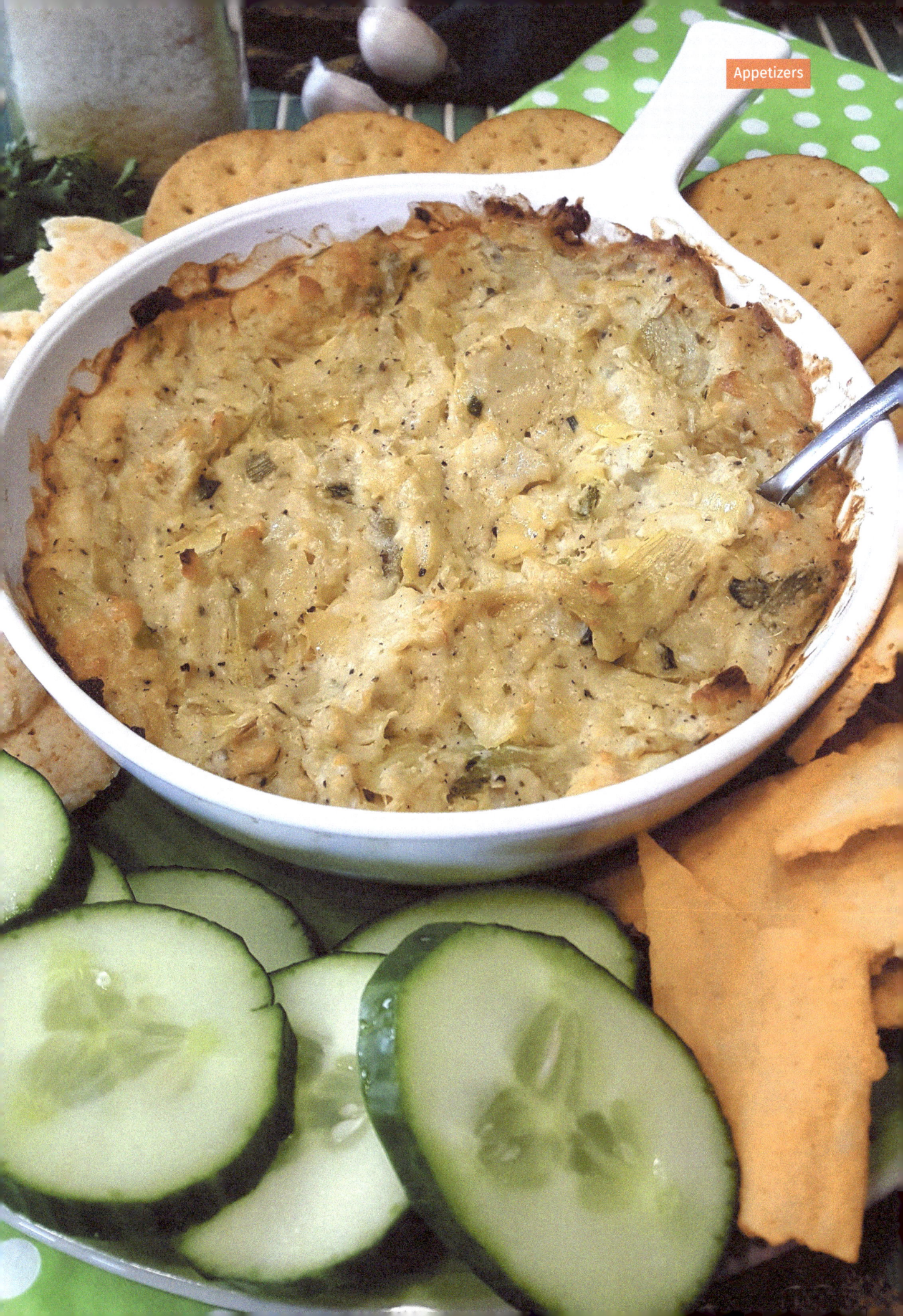

Appetizers

CRAB CAKES

These crab cakes are tender and refreshing. They could also make a great lunch option with a side salad.

INGREDIENTS

Makes eight crab cakes

- 3 T. half-fat mayonnaise (I use Hellman's)
- 2 t. Dijon mustard
- 2 T. egg (scramble egg, then measure)
- 2 green onions, finely minced
- ½ t. seafood seasoning (I use Old Bay)
- 1 lb. lump or jumbo lump crab (may use drained canned)
- 1 T. unsalted butter
- A squeeze of fresh lemon

INSTRUCTIONS

Pre-heat oven to 400°F.

1. Blend mayonnaise, mustard, egg, onions, and Old Bay in a large bowl.
2. Gently fold in the crab, being careful not to break up the lumps too much (make sure to discard any pieces of shell or spongy bits that you see).
3. Using a large scoop, divide into eight even portions on a parchment or foil-lined baking sheet.
4. Drizzle a few drops of melted butter on top of each cake. Bake 20 to 25 minutes, until lightly browned. Add a squeeze of lemon before serving, and a dollop of this wonderful tartar sauce below.

QUICK TARTAR SAUCE (RECIPE MAY BE DOUBLED)

Mix the following in a small bowl:

- 1 T. half-fat mayonnaise
- 2 T. plain Greek yogurt
- ½ t. Dijon mustard
- 1 t. onion, minced
- 1 t. lemon juice
- 1 T. bread and butter pickles, minced (recipe found in the Sides)
- Salt and ground black pepper to taste
- A pinch of granular sweetener

NOTE: If you are using canned crab, just be aware it is usually very salty and I find it yields a salty crab cake. Ideally, if you can find low-sodium, or, better yet, salt-free, that would be better.

Appetizers

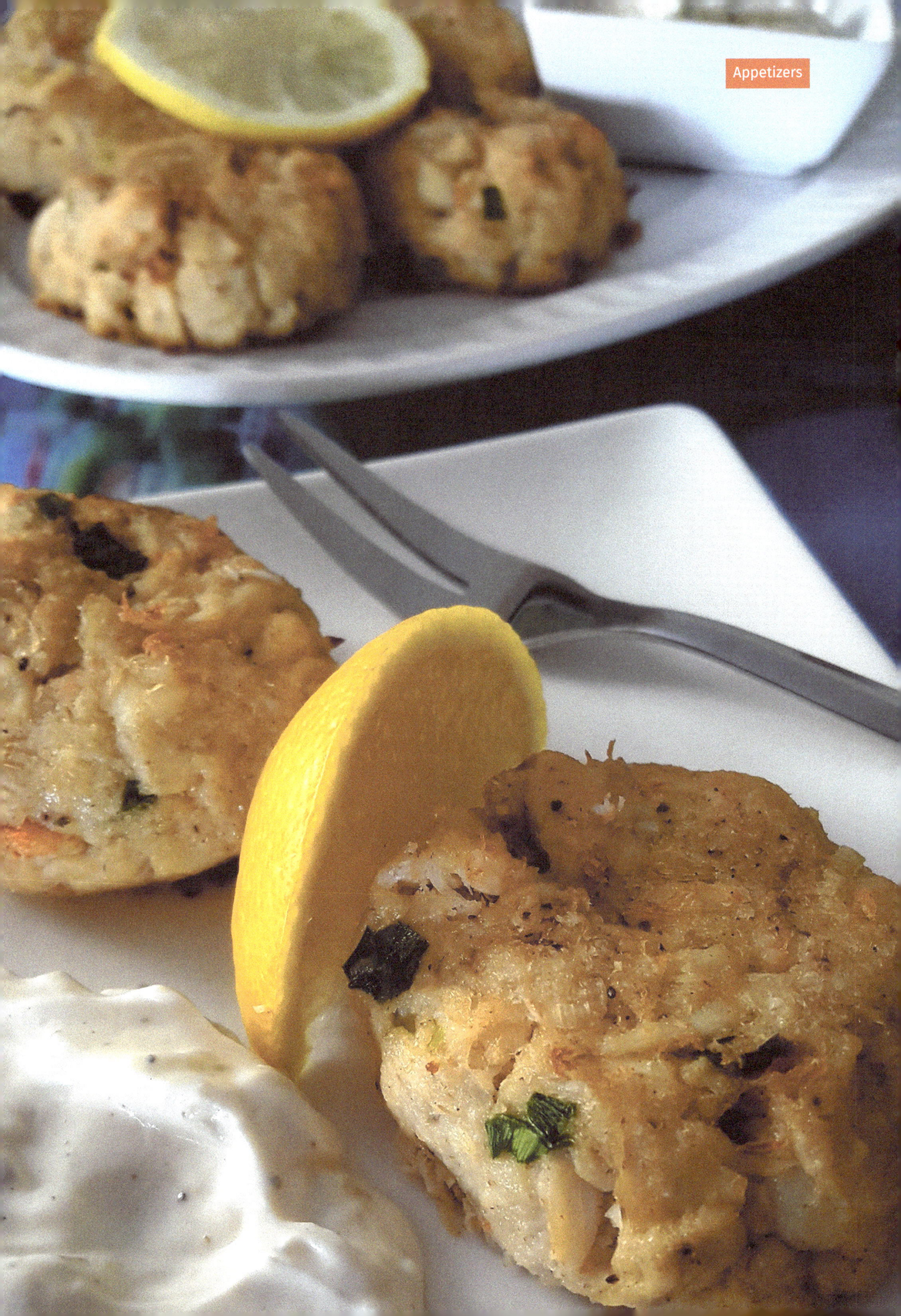

ITALIAN CHICKEN AND ZUCCHINI POPPERS

These are moist and delectable bites with all-Italian flavour. They are extremely easy to prepare and will be a favourite in your house. I like to eat a few as a light lunch. The warm marinara sauce for dipping adds an extra layer of comfort.

INGREDIENTS

- 1 T. olive oil
- 8 oz. chicken breast, chopped into fine chunks, not ground (do this while still half frozen)
- 1 medium zucchini, shredded and drained
- 2 cloves garlic, minced
- 2 heaping T. parmesan
- 1½ t. dried Italian spice blend
- ½ t. salt
- ½ t. ground black pepper
- 1 T. panko bread crumbs
- ½ egg (beat it then measure)

INSTRUCTIONS

1. In a medium-sized bowl, combine all the ingredients except for the oil.
2. Shape into small patties using about one-quarter cup of the mixture for each (use a measuring cup as a guide) until the mixture is gone.
3. Using a non-stick skillet, heat the olive oil over medium heat and add the patties to the skillet.
4. Cook the patties three to four minutes per side, then flip gently and continue to cook for another three to four minutes until golden and cooked thoroughly through.
5. Plate the patties and sprinkle them with parmesan cheese.
6. Serve with warmed low-sugar marinara sauce from the jar or homemade.

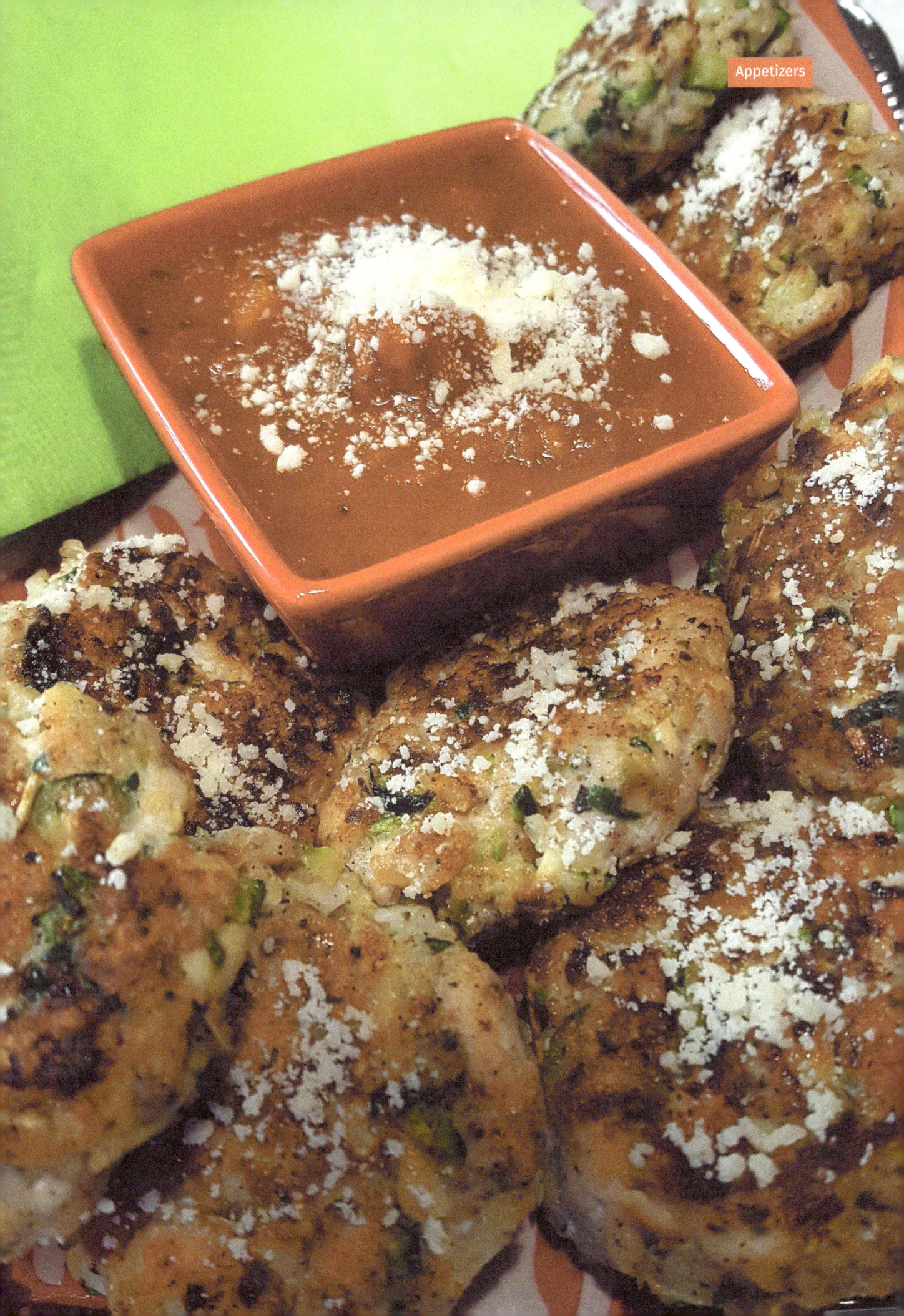

Appetizers

COMFORT COOKING
for Bariatric Post-Ops and Everyone Else!

BUFFALO WING CHICKEN BALLS

I remember the days when I never thought twice about ordering wings as an appetizer or a large basket as a main dish. Those times are in the past and now we can still have the taste of a great buffalo wing without the guilt. This one is moist, spicy, and just plain delicious.

INGREDIENTS

- Vegetable cooking spray
- 1½ lb. ground chicken
- 1 T. olive oil
- ¼ c. panko bread crumbs
- ¼ c. parmesan cheese
- ¼ c. celery, finely chopped
- ½ c. onion, finely chopped
- 1 egg
- 1 t. salt
- 1 t. garlic powder
- ¼ t. ground black pepper
- ½ c. hot sauce (I use Frank's)
- 1 T. butter (melted)
- low-calorie, low-sugar blue cheese dressing (I use Bolthouse Farms blue cheese yogurt dressing)

INSTRUCTIONS

1. In a medium-sized bowl, mix all the ingredients together except for the hot sauce, butter, and the blue cheese dressing. Combine well and shape into mini balls. Tip: Spray your hands with cooking spray before shaping the balls, otherwise you will have a sticky mess.

2. Using a large skillet sprayed with cooking spray, add the olive oil and heat up to medium heat. Add the chicken balls and cook till lightly browned and no longer pink inside. Flip the balls to make sure all sides are browned evenly. Remove from heat and transfer to a glass bowl.

3. In another small bowl or cup, combine the hot sauce and the melted butter and stir well. Pour the sauce over the chicken balls and stir gently to distribute evenly.

4. To serve, arrange balls on a serving platter with celery sticks and toothpicks nearby.

5. Pour out about one-half cup of the blue cheese dressing into a small dish and place next to the chicken balls for dipping. Enjoy!

Appetizers

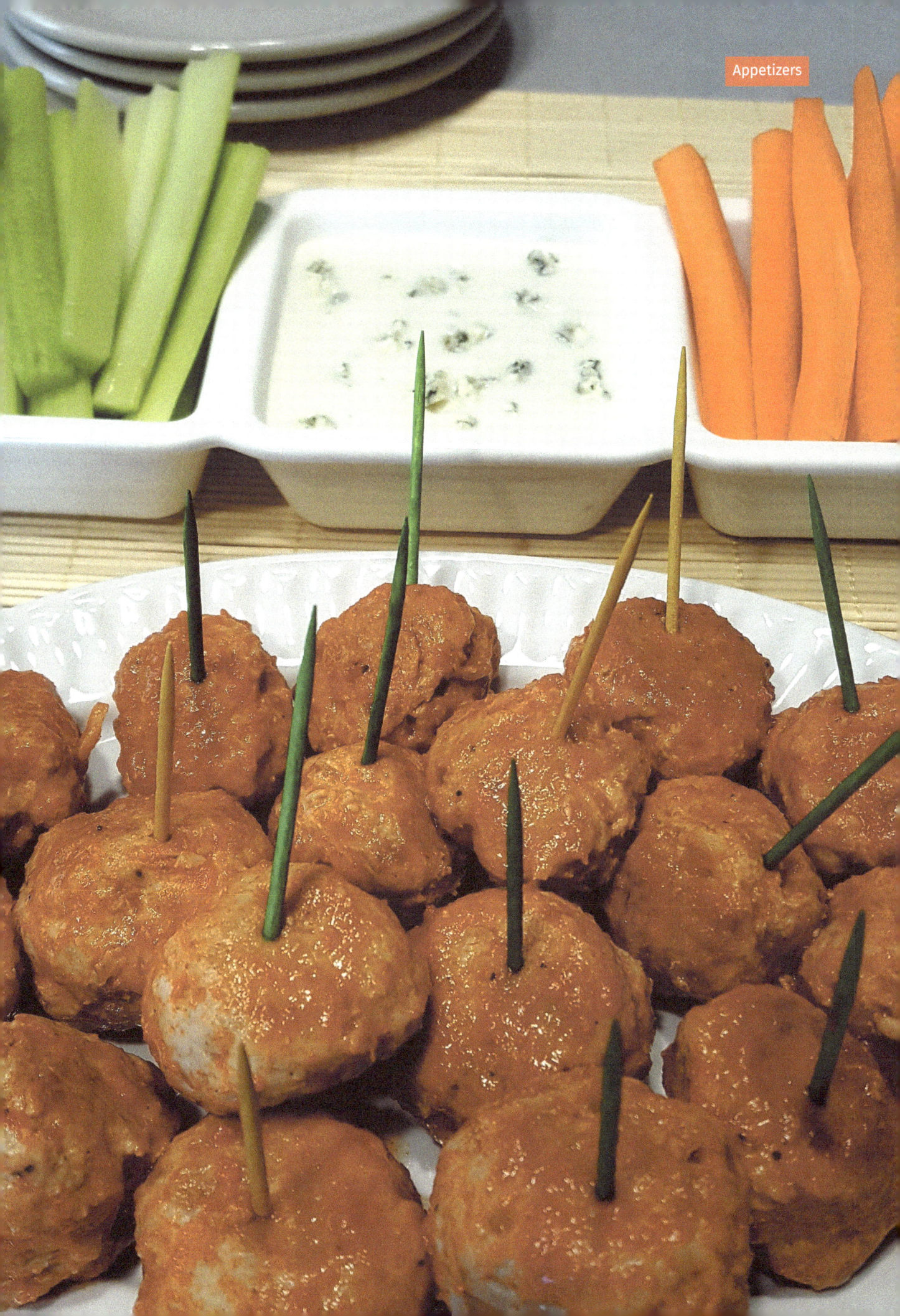

COMFORT COOKING
for Bariatric Post-Ops and Everyone Else!

TERIYAKI WINGS ON A SKEWER

We don't partake in regular wings anymore, so here's a tasty way to enjoy the teriyaki flavours. The sesame seed oil is an absolute must, so do not omit it or substitute with another oil. This is a great recipe to use in the summer months on the grill or any time during the year.

INGREDIENTS

- 10 chicken tenders (season with salt and pepper)
- 1 T. olive oil
- Vegetable cooking spray
- ⅔ c. soy sauce
- 2 T. sesame seed oil
- ⅓ c. white vinegar
- ⅓ c. no-added-sugar orange preserves (I use Smucker's)
- ½ t. salt
- ¼ t. black pepper
- 1 T. Truvia Brown Sugar Blend
- 10 bamboo skewers, soaked in water and patted dry

INSTRUCTIONS

1. Measure the skewers and make sure they are short enough to fit into your skillet. If they are too long then snip them. They will be easy to shorten if they have been soaking in water. Ignore this step if you are grilling them on your BBQ.

2. In a small pot, combine the soy sauce, sesame seed oil, vinegar, orange preserves, salt, pepper, and Truvia Brown Sugar Blend. Warm the mixture up over low heat but do not boil. Stir well and divide the sauce into one large bowl and one small bowl.

3. Add the chicken to the large bowl, making sure that all parts are immersed in the marinade. Cover with plastic wrap and place in the fridge for one hour. Cover the small bowl with plastic wrap and place in the fridge until ready to prepare.

4. Remove the chicken after the one hour and start to thread the chicken through the dried bamboo skewers.

5. Using a large skillet sprayed with cooking spray, add the olive oil and heat up to medium. Arrange the first five skewers into the pan and cook for two to three minutes per side. When the chicken is no longer pink, remove the skewers to a shallow dish. Continue cooking the last five.

6. Drizzle the remaining sauce (small bowl) over the chicken.

Appetizers

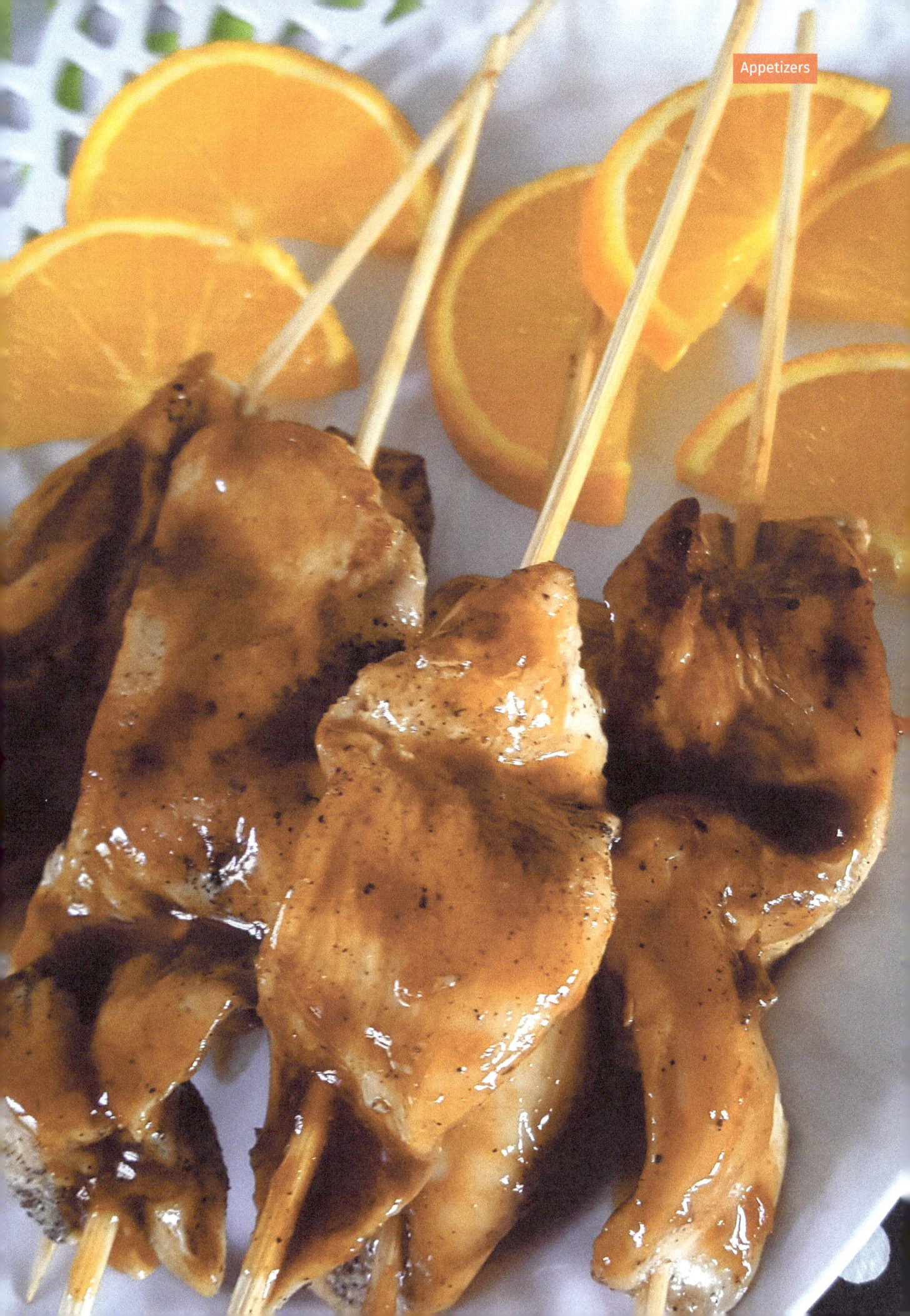

HUMMUS

You can purchase hummus anywhere now as it is found in every store on the planet. However, this recipe is so good and so simple that you may never buy commercial again!

INGREDIENTS

16 oz. can chick peas, drained

¼ c. tahini paste OR smooth peanut butter

¼ c. or more fresh lemon juice

3 garlic cloves

½ t. sea salt

½ t. ground cumin

¼ t. black pepper

2 T. olive oil (reserve 1 T. for the garnish)

Dash of paprika for garnish

½ c. warm water

INSTRUCTIONS

1. In a food processor, combine chick peas, tahini or peanut butter, lemon juice, garlic, salt, cumin, pepper, and one tablespoon olive oil—process until smooth.

2. Scrape down sides of bowl. Process again, pouring in one-half cup warm water until hummus is smooth.

3. Transfer to a serving bowl and drizzle about one tablespoon of olive oil over top and a sprinkle of paprika. Eat with a spoon or dip with vegetables!

Appetizers

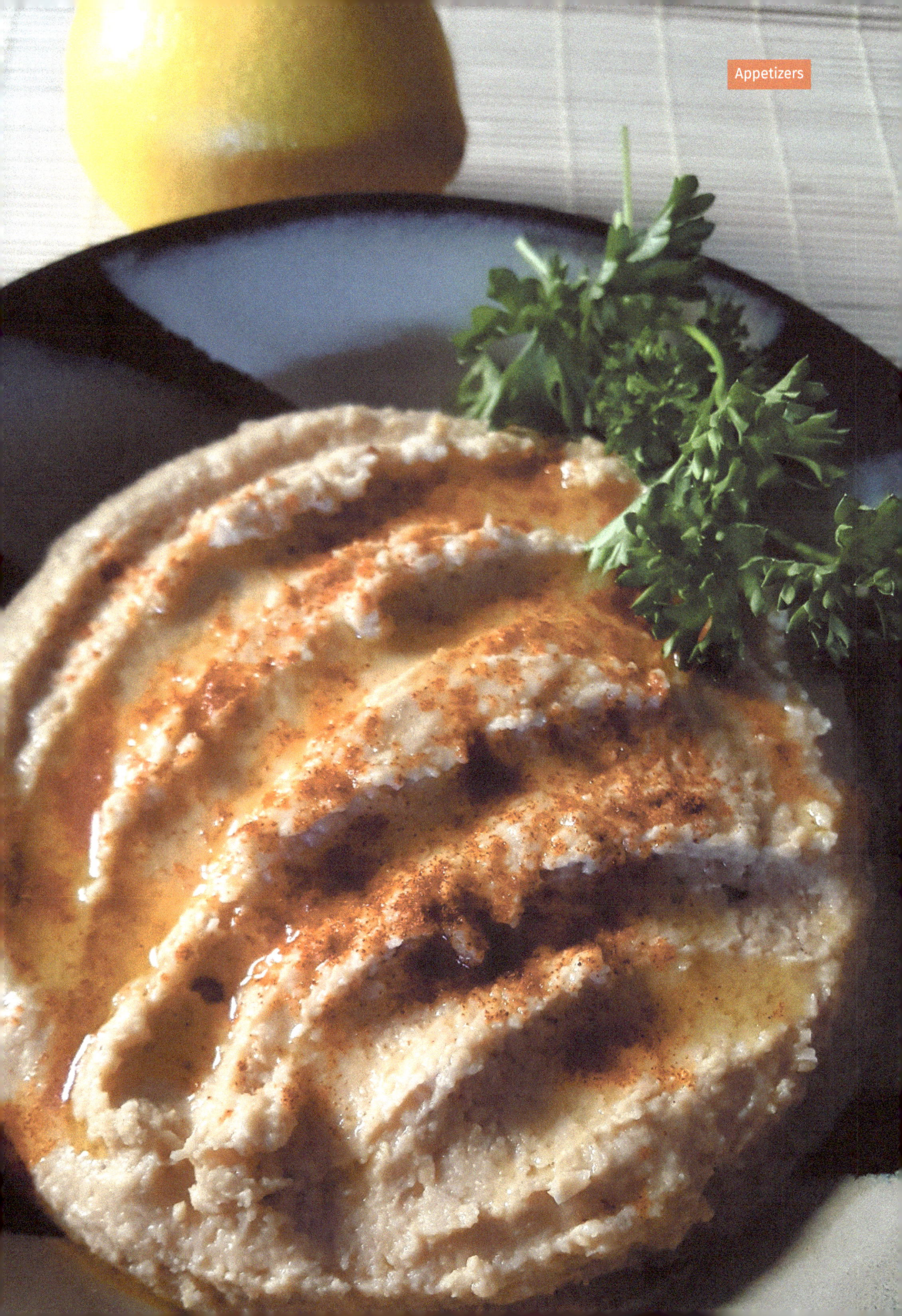

COMFORT COOKING
for Bariatric Post-Ops and Everyone Else!

YUMMY GUACAMOLE

Who doesn't love avocados, and this is the best guacamole ever! I like to eat this with a spoon or as a dip with red peppers.

INGREDIENTS

- 3 soft and ripened avocados (I use the Hass variety)
- Juice of 1 lime
- 1 t. half-fat mayonnaise (I use Hellmann's)
- 2 Roma tomatoes, cut in half and diced
- 2 garlic cloves, mashed with a garlic press
- ½ t. tabasco
- Kosher salt and pepper

INSTRUCTIONS

1. Mash avocados in a large bowl with a fork, leaving mixture slightly chunky. Fold in lime juice, tomatoes, mayonnaise, and garlic.
2. Season with salt, black pepper, and tabasco to taste. Serve immediately.

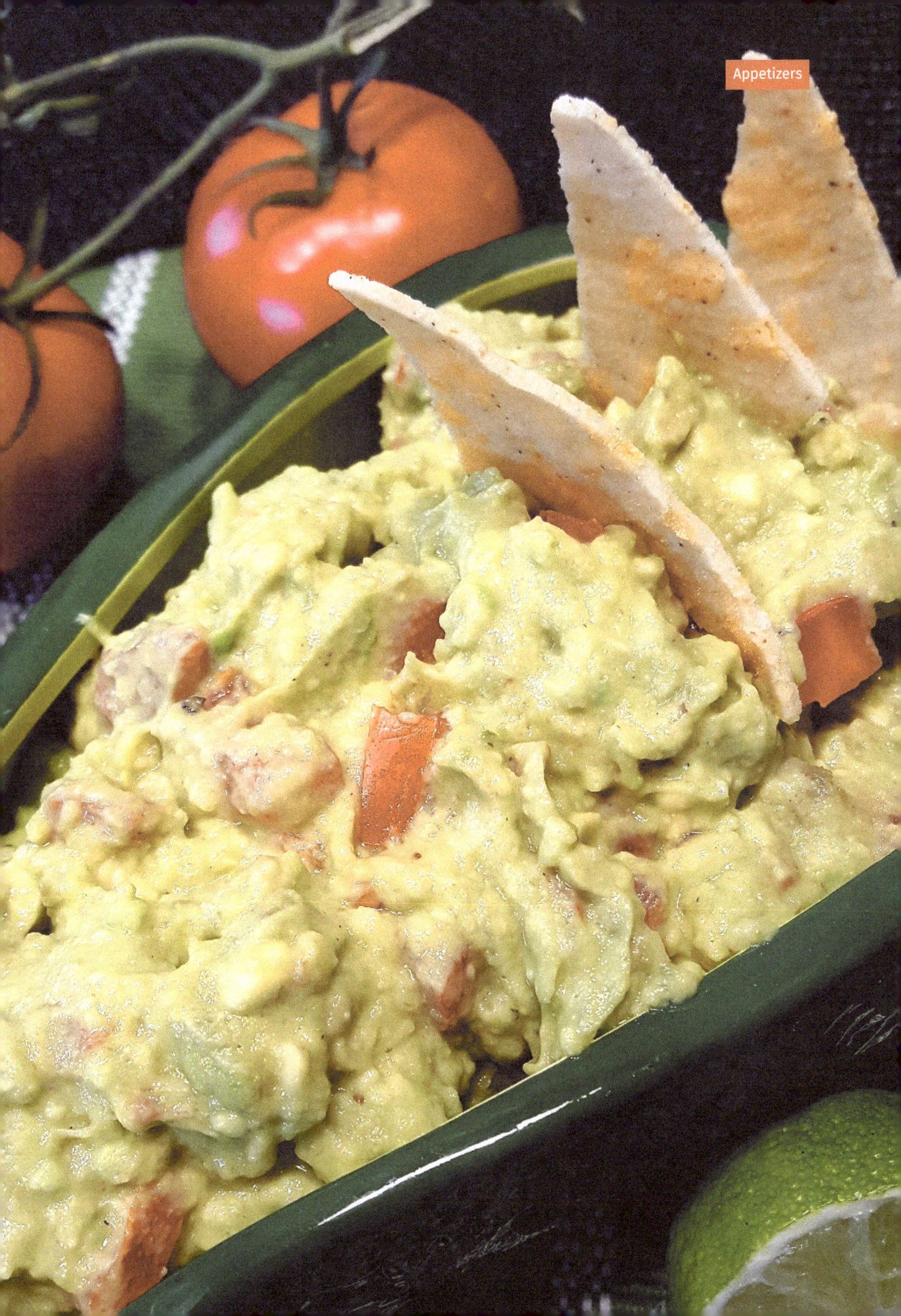

Appetizers

CURRIED DEVILLED EGGS

Delicious, nutritious, and looks lovely on an appetizer table. You can halve the recipe and keep these in the fridge to have as a great protein snack any time of day. If you don't like curry spice then omit if you wish.

INGREDIENTS

- 12 eggs, hard-boiled
- ⅓ c. 0% plain Greek yogurt
- ⅓ c. half-fat mayonnaise (I use Hellman's)
- ½ t. curry powder (optional)
- 1 t. Dijon mustard
- ½ t. sea salt or less
- Fresh ground black pepper
- Smoked paprika as garnish

INSTRUCTIONS

1. Cut the eggs in half lengthwise.
2. Scoop out the yolks into a small bowl. Add the yogurt, mayonnaise, curry powder, mustard, salt, and pepper. Mash with a fork until smooth and mixed well.
3. Arrange the egg whites on a large serving platter. Spoon or pipe filling into egg whites and garnish with paprika.

Appetizers

STUFFED MUSHROOMS

When deciding which appetizers to make, you must include these. They are very easy to make, and the protein replaces the package of cream cheese and cups of bread crumbs!

INGREDIENTS

- 1 T. olive oil
- 12 large stuffing mushroom caps, stems removed, chopped and reserved
- Sea salt and ground black pepper
- 6 oz. Italian or regular sausage
- 3 cloves garlic, chopped finely
- 1 small onion, chopped finely
- ¼ c. red pepper, minced
- ¼ c. parsley, chopped
- ¼ c. panko bread crumbs
- ¼ c. parmesan cheese
- 2 T. light cream cheese

INSTRUCTIONS

1. In a large skillet, heat up oil over medium heat and sauté mushroom caps, smooth side down, for three to four minutes until browned and liquid collects in the caps.

2. Flip them over and brown the edges of the cup side for one to two minutes. Remove from the skillet and set on a paper towel to drain.

3. Over medium heat, brown the sausage and the chopped mushroom stems in the same skillet, mashing the meat as it cooks to smooth out the texture. Pour off any fat from the pan then add the garlic, onion and red pepper, continuing to cook until they are softened and dried (about 10 minutes).

4. Remove from heat and allow to cool slightly.

5. Add the parsley, breadcrumbs, and cheeses. Season with salt and pepper to taste.

6. Arrange mushroom caps, cup side up, on a baking sheet prepared with parchment paper. Using a spoon, pack each mushroom with the mixture, rounding and smoothing the tops so they all look uniform.

7. Cover in foil and bake at 400°F for 10 to 12 minutes until bubbly. Remove the foil and bake an additional five minutes to brown.

Appetizers

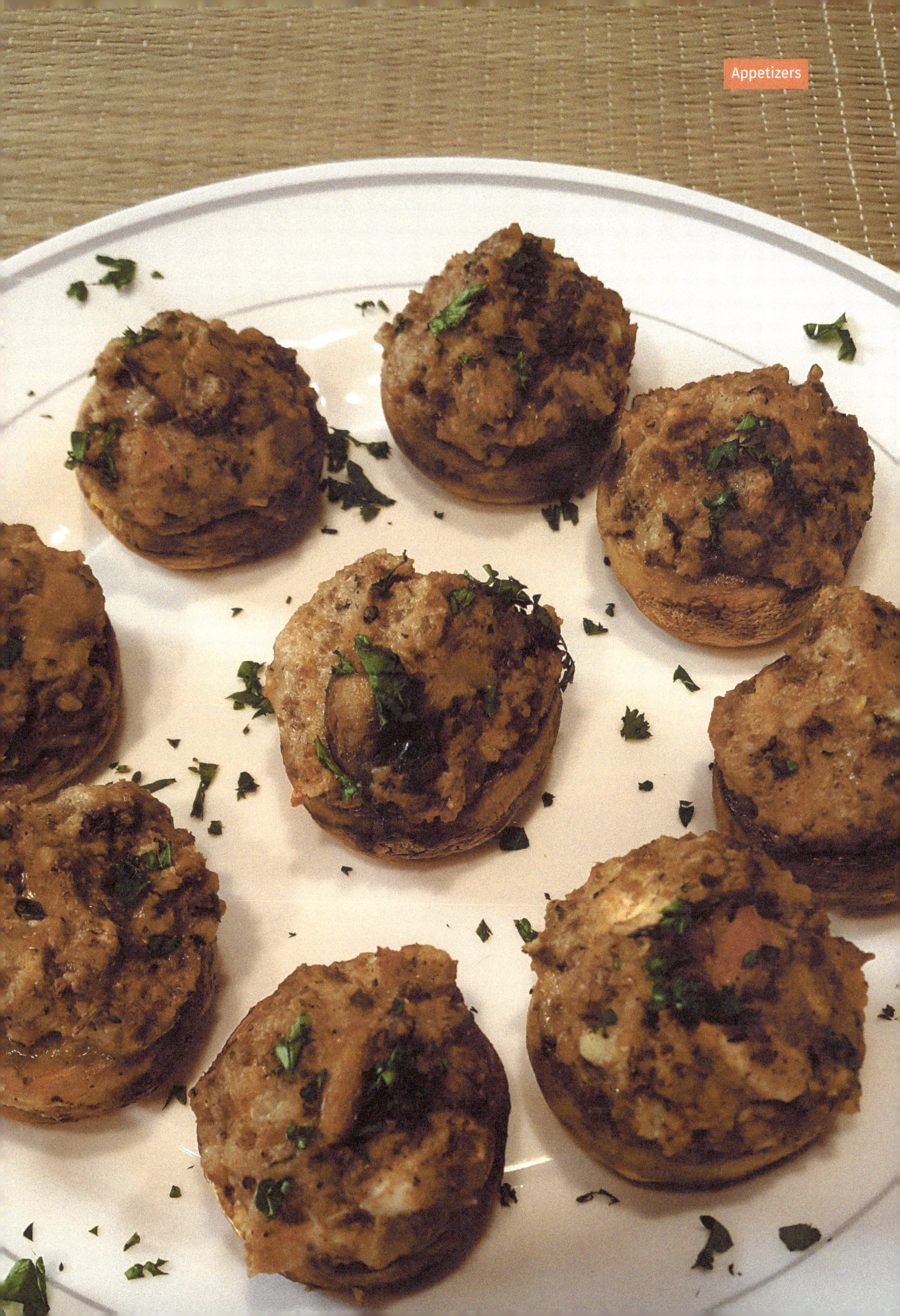

CHEESE AND CHIVES BROWNIES

These are simply yummy. If you are wondering what you can bring to a party, this is it! Makes 25 to 36 bite-sized squares.

INGREDIENTS

8 oz. reduced-fat cheddar cheese, shredded
1 medium jalapeno pepper, chopped finely
½ c. milk
¼ c. flour
3 large eggs

½ t. sea salt
¼ t. black pepper
½ t. onion powder
1 t. hot sauce (I use Sriracha)
3 T. green onion or chives, chopped

INSTRUCTIONS

Pre-heat oven to 325°F.

1. Spray an 8 × 8-inch square glass oven dish with cooking spray.
2. Arrange the cheese evenly in the dish, adding the peppers and onion on top.
3. In a bowl, combine the milk, flour, eggs, salt, pepper, onion powder, and hot sauce until smooth.
4. Slowly pour over the cheese. Bake for 25 to 30 minutes till browned and puffed. Do not overbake. The centre should jiggle when you take it out of the oven. Cut when slightly warm but not cool.
5. Serve with salsa or eat them plain.

Appetizers

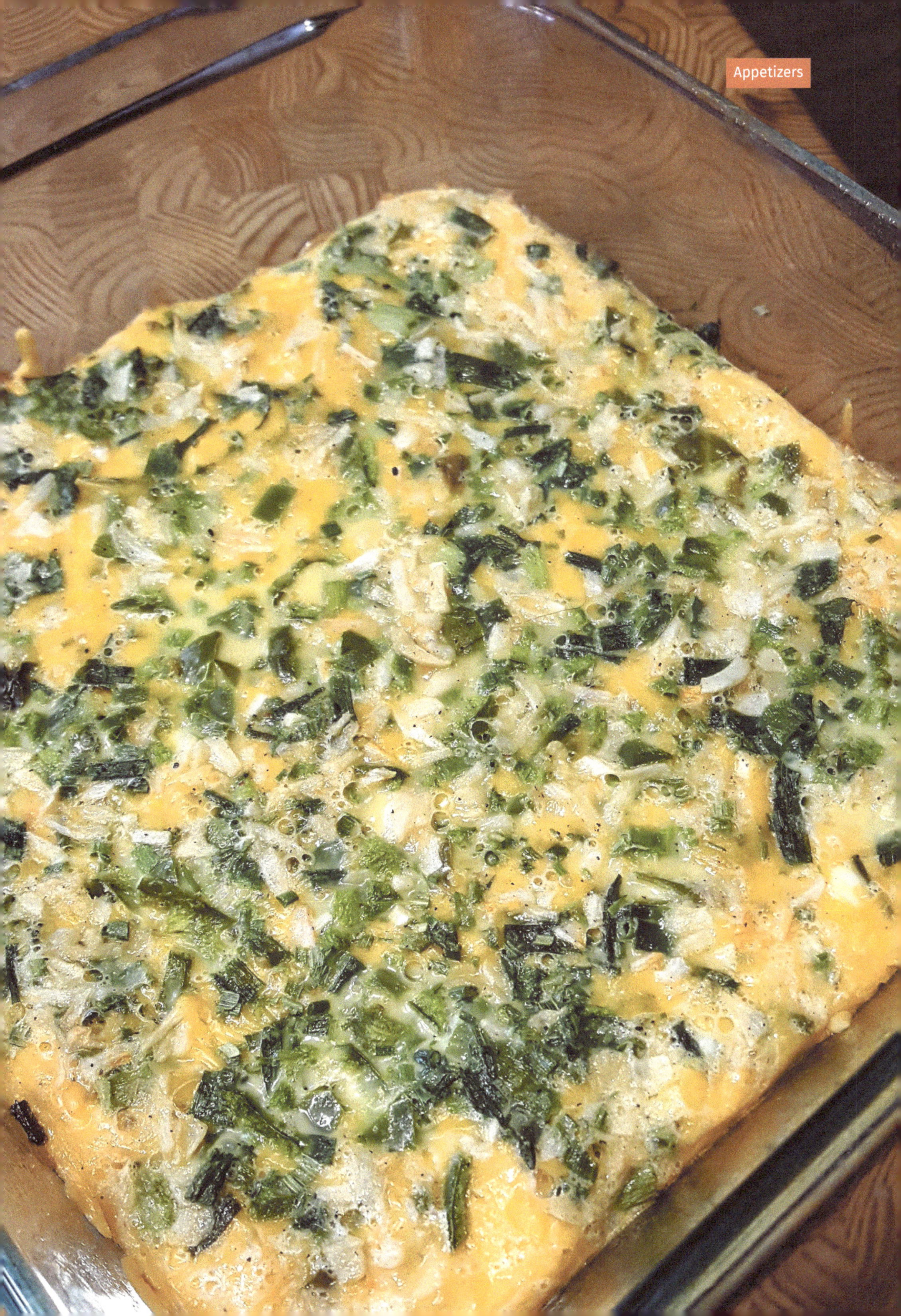

COMFORT COOKING
for Bariatric Post-Ops and Everyone Else!

MINI QUICHES

For breakfast or lunch, these mini quiches are soft, squishy, and delicious! If having them for lunch, pair with a nice green side salad and low-carb dressing.

INGREDIENTS

1 t. olive oil

1 t. butter

1 medium onion, diced

1 c. mushrooms, chopped

1 c. frozen chopped spinach (thawed and squeezed dry)

¼ c. red peppers, diced

½ c. bacon, sausage, or ham, cooked and crumbled (optional but if making a breakfast quiche you might want to add. Totally up to you.)

¼ t. garlic powder

¼ t. paprika

¼ t. black pepper

¼ t. salt

Pinch of nutmeg

⅓ c. baking mix (I use Bisquick original baking mix)

1 c. milk (I use ½ c. 1% milk and ½ c. unsweetened almond milk)

2 eggs

4 oz. reduced fat cheddar cheese, shredded (shred your own. It's less expensive and doesn't have the chemicals found in bagged shredded cheese.)

INSTRUCTIONS

Pre-heat oven to 400°F and spray 12 muffin tins with non-stick cooking spray.

1. In a skillet, add olive oil and butter and heat to medium–high, until bubbly. Reduce heat to medium–low and add the onions, cooking for two to three minutes.

2. Add the red pepper and mushrooms and cook for two minutes until they start to release liquid. Add the spinach, crumbled cooked bacon, and all spices. Continue to cook until tender.

3. Remove from heat and let cool slightly. Place a heaping tablespoon of the mixture into each muffin tin.

4. In a medium-sized bowl, combine Bisquick, milk, and eggs until well blended. Stir in the cheese. Carefully ladle enough batter mixture onto each muffin tin, not quite to the top. Repeat until each mini quiche is complete.

5. Bake for approximately 15 to 17 minutes, until quiche appear puffy. Centre should be cooked through but slightly loose. Do not overbake, otherwise the quiche will have a dried texture.

6. Remove from oven and allow them to cool for five minutes before removing them carefully. These may be kept in the freezer and heated up individually in the microwave.

Appetizers

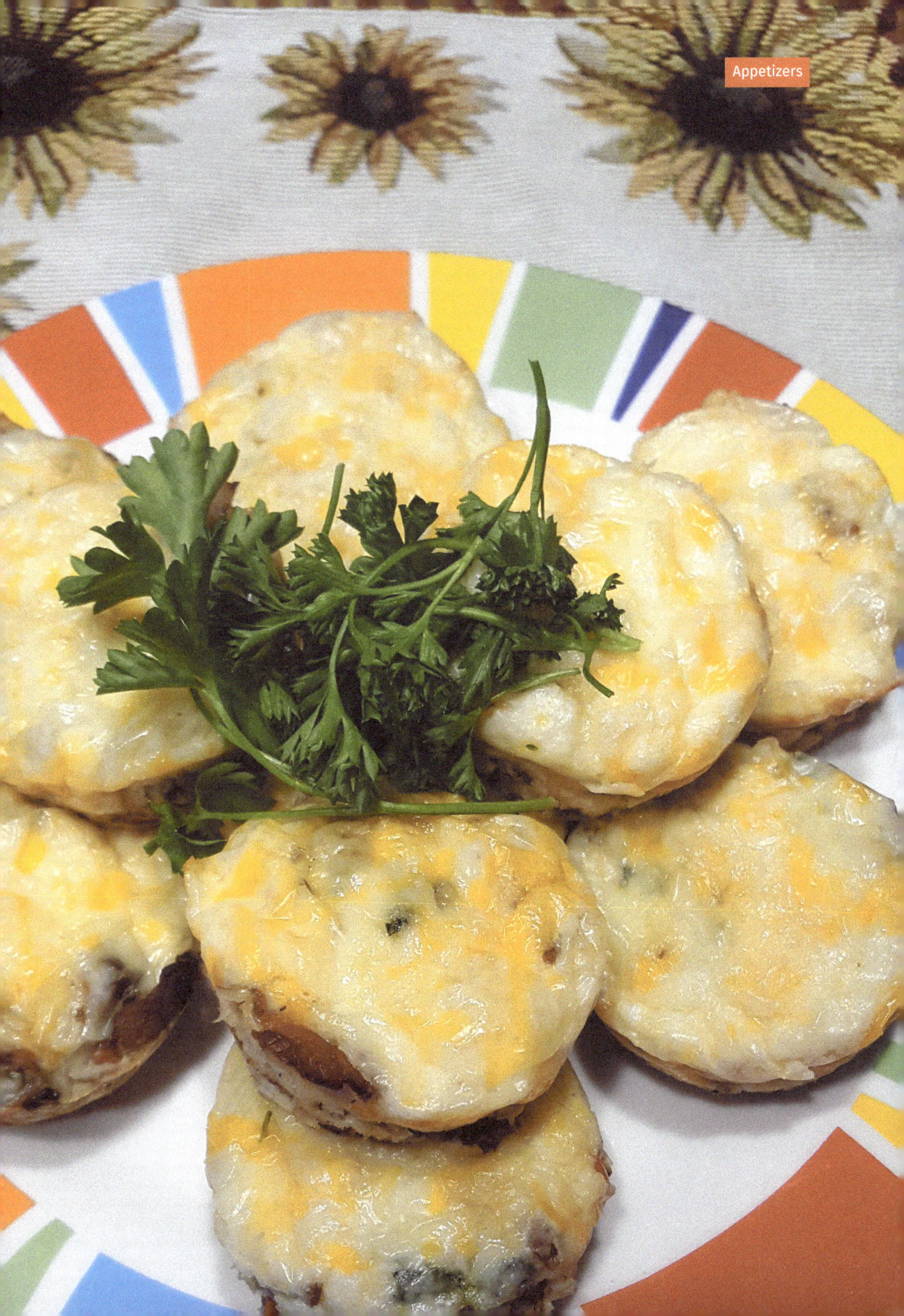

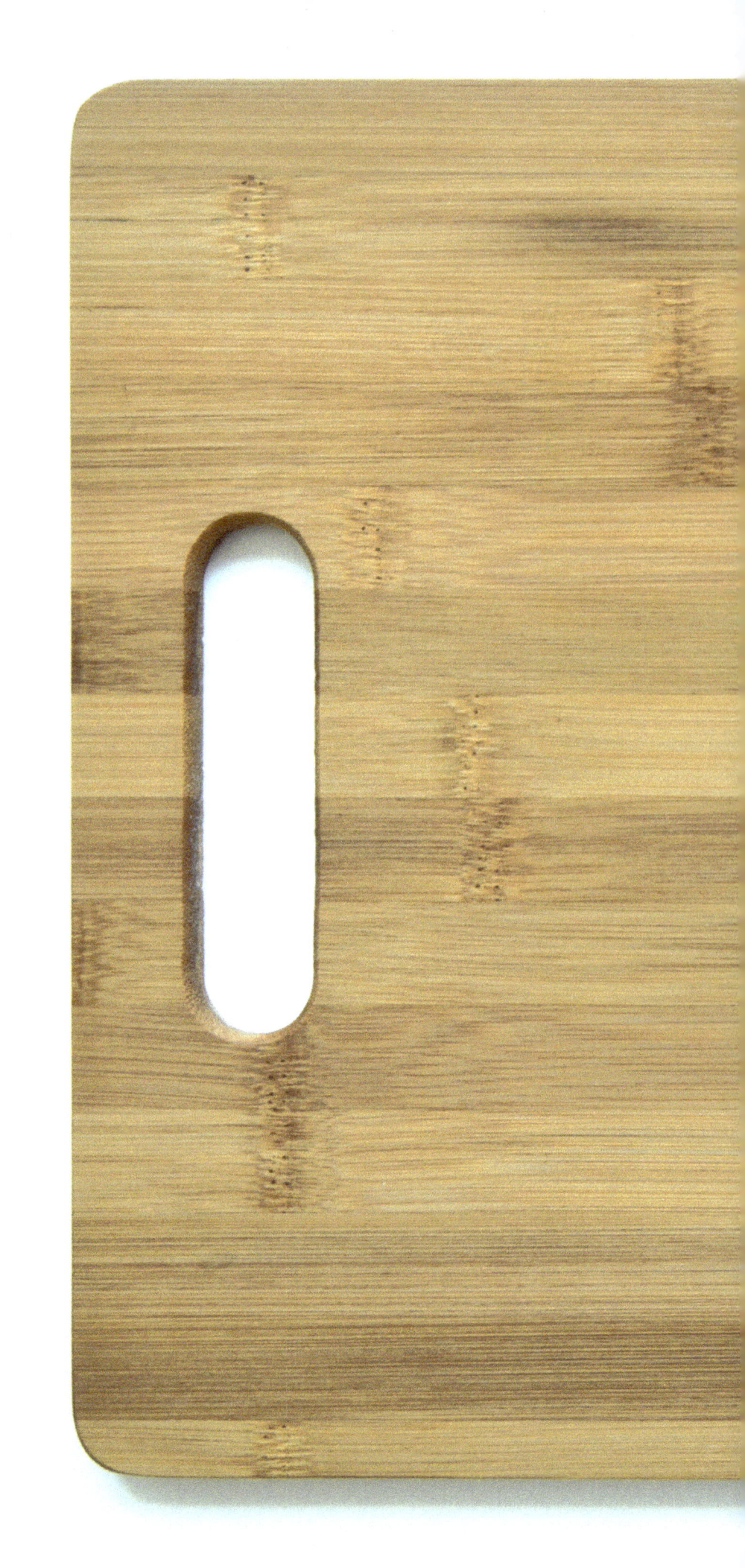

BEVERAGES

Delicious Hot Cocoa Mix 38

Cranberry Cider. 40

Strawberry Lemonade 42

Skinny Mocha Frappé. 44

Sugar-Free Holiday Eggnog! 46

DELICIOUS HOT COCOA MIX

This is my go-to beverage in the winter. A must-have treat when the wind is howling and you need an instant warmup. This recipe makes about 10 cups but can be easily doubled to ensure hot cocoa any time!

INGREDIENTS

- 1 c. Truvia Baking Blend
- 1 c. dark unsweetened cocoa powder
- 2½ c. powdered low fat milk
- 1 t. salt
- 2 t. cornstarch
- ½ t. ground cinnamon
- Pinch of cayenne pepper (optional)

INSTRUCTIONS

1. Whisk all the ingredients in a large bowl and combine well. Store in an airtight container.

To serve: Add about three tablespoons of powder to a mug. Add one cup of boiled water. Tastes will vary so if you feel it's too sweet then add more water or if it's not sweet enough then add a touch more cocoa powder. Stir well to blend. I sometimes add a splash of sugar-free, non-dairy coffee creamer; however, this is optional. For something extra-special, add a dollop of sugar-free whipped cream or regular Cool Whip!

SEASONAL FLAVOURS

For gingerbread cocoa: Measure out three tablespoons of powder in a mug, one-quarter teaspoon ground cinnamon, one-quarter teaspoon ground nutmeg, a pinch of ground cloves, and a pinch of ground ginger. Add the boiled water and stir until well blended. Enjoy!

For pumpkin pie cocoa: Add to the three tablespoons of powder, one-half teaspoon pumpkin spice, plus one tablespoon pumpkin puree (not pie filling).

For peanut butter cup cocoa: Add to the three tablespoons of powder, two tablespoons peanut butter powder and pour in the boiled water.

For coconut or mint flavour: Add one-quarter teaspoon of flavoured extract after adding the boiled water and stir.

NOTE: If you are not whipping up your own sugar-free whipped cream then you can use sugar-free Cool Whip.

Beverages

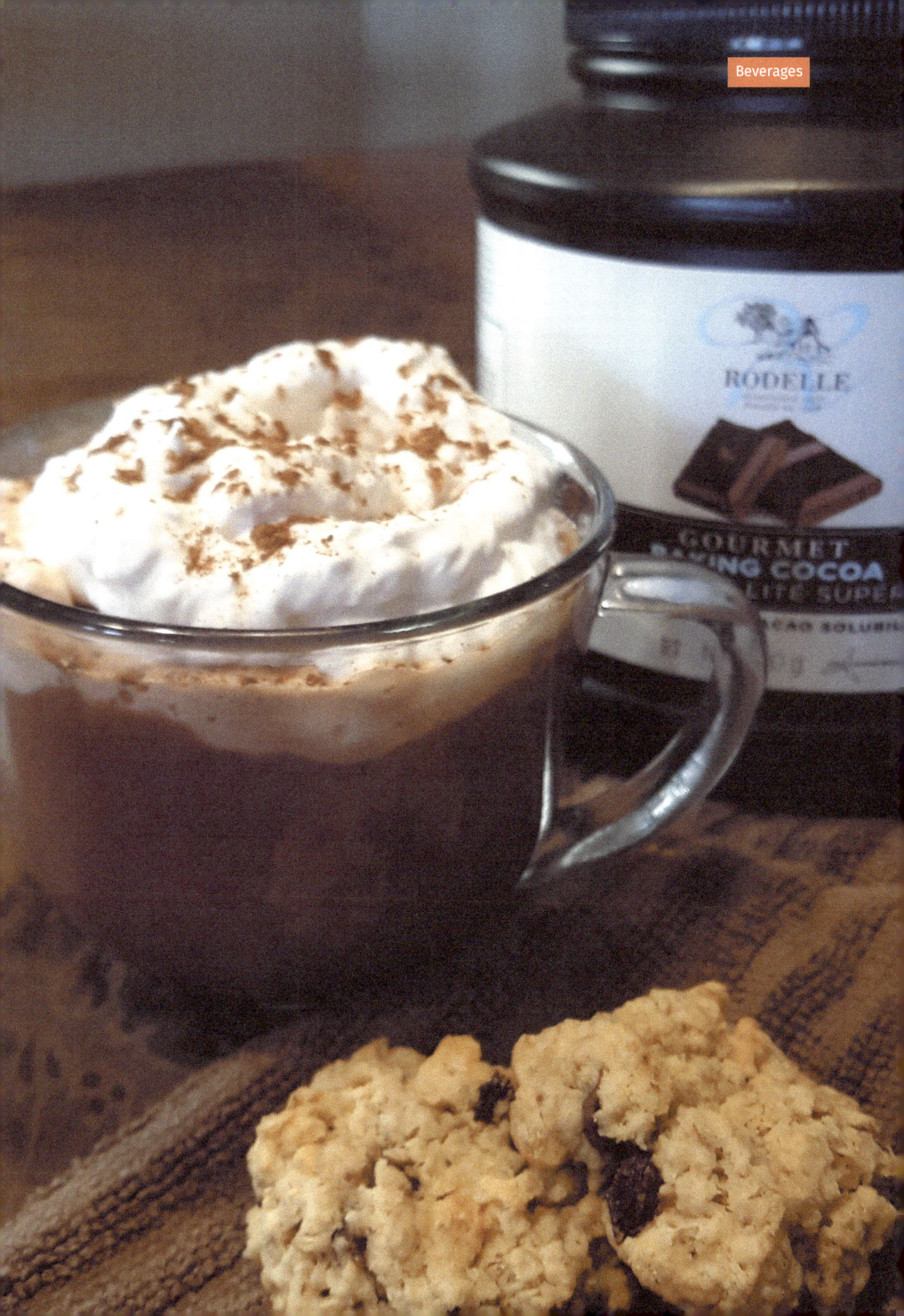

CRANBERRY CIDER

This is one of those great fall drinks that will warm your insides when there is a chill in the air.

INGREDIENTS

¼ c. Truvia Baking Blend
2 cinnamon sticks
10 whole cloves
¼ t. ground nutmeg

6 c. diet cranberry juice (I use Ocean Spray sweetened with Splenda)
1 medium orange, washed and sliced in half

INSTRUCTIONS

1. Combine Truvia, spices, and diet cranberry juice in a pot.
2. Cut orange in half, squeeze the juice into pot, and add the peel in with the rest of the ingredients.
3. Simmer over low heat for 15 minutes. Do not boil. Remove cinnamon sticks, cloves, and peel.
4. Serve in glass mugs and garnish with a slice of orange. I like it tart so I add about one tablespoon of lemon juice to my glass mug. Delicious!

Beverages

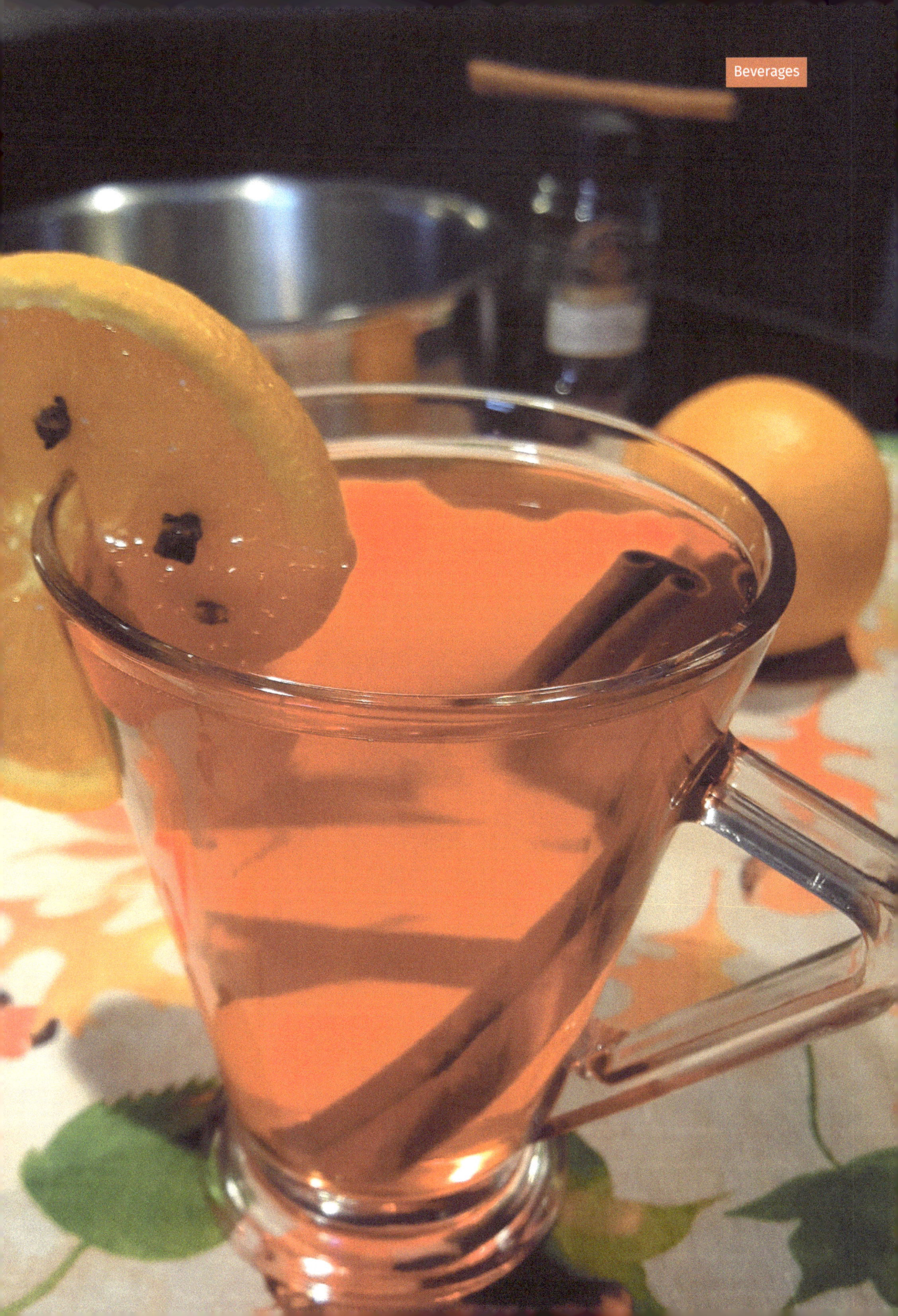

STRAWBERRY LEMONADE

Nothing beats a cold glass of fruit-infused lemonade in hot weather. This recipe is one of the easiest!

INGREDIENTS

- 2 packets (1 pitcher each) sugar-free lemonade drink mix (I use Crystal Light)
- 8 c. cold water
- 6–8 frozen strawberries

INSTRUCTIONS

1. In a nice glass pitcher, add the drink mix and water. Mix well and add the frozen berries. Place in the fridge to allow the flavours and colours to develop as it chills, preferably overnight. Serve over ice with a lemon slice.

Note: Be daring! Add sprigs of mint, rosemary, ginger, or lavender to kick up the flavours. Remember to remove the sprigs before serving!

Beverages

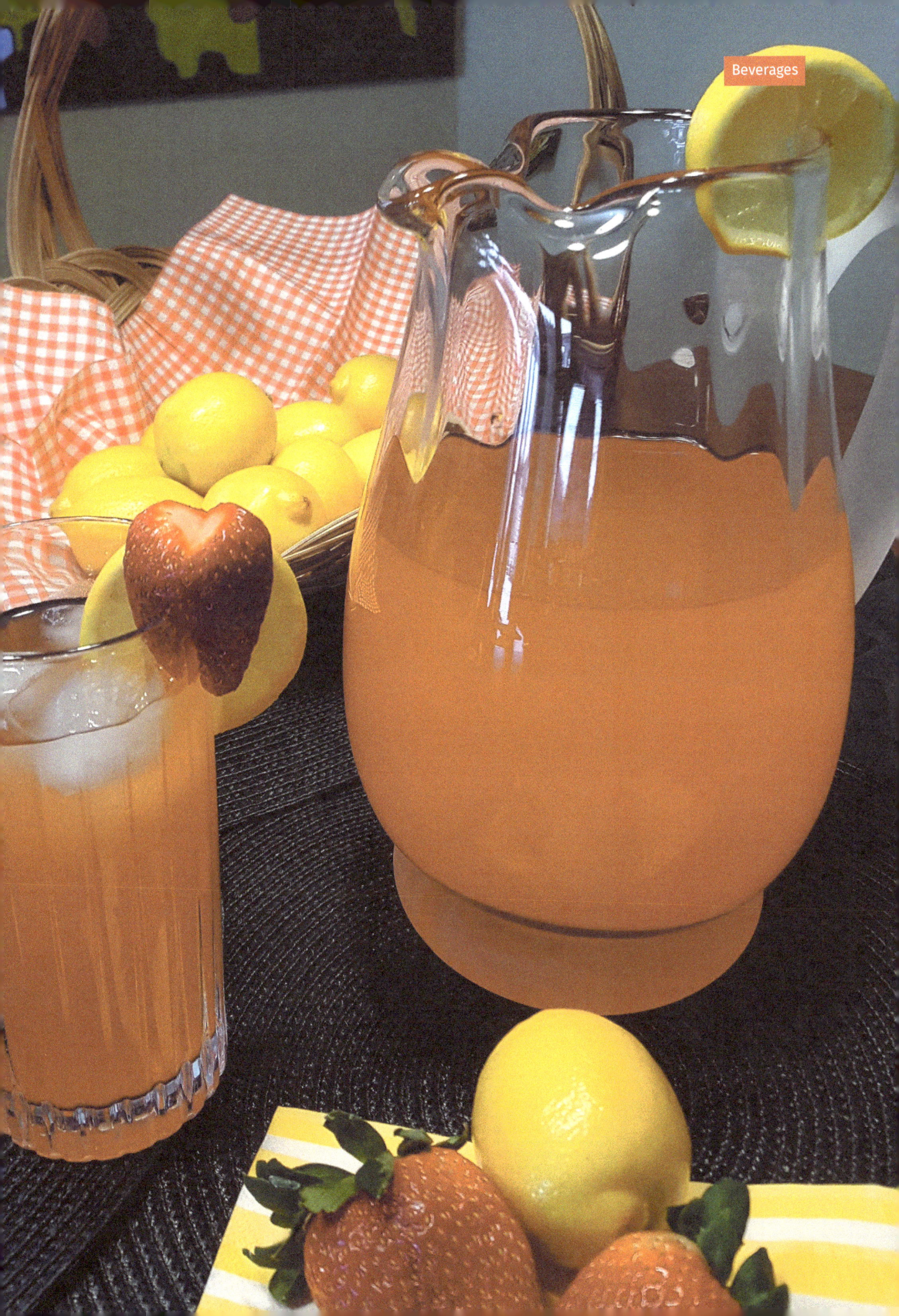

SKINNY MOCHA FRAPPÉ

The trendy coffee industry has exploded all over the world, and has even made its way into the fast-food market. You can get practically every kind of coffee drink anywhere at any time; however, they are mostly sugar bombs and very expensive. I know people who must have their daily fix, and for them, the money saved by making it at home could send them on a yearly vacation! For iced coffee lovers, here is a tasty cool treat made with the ingredients you already have in your kitchen. You can even add in a scoop of chocolate protein powder and make it a summer breakfast or afternoon snack!

INGREDIENTS

Serves two

- 1 c. extra-strong brewed coffee, cold (you may use regular or decaf)
- 3 t. instant coffee granules
- 2 T. sugar-free vanilla or chocolate syrup (such as Torani)
- ½ c. 1 % milk
- 3 T. hot cocoa mix powder (Delicious Hot Chocolate Mix recipe in this section)
- 2½ t. Truvia Baking Blend
- 1½ T. sugar-free chocolate pudding powder
- Few grains sea salt
- 3 T. sugar-free Cool Whip
- 3 T. sugar-free vanilla coffee whitener (I use International Delight)
- 2½–3 c. party ice (small, clear cubes)

INSTRUCTIONS

1. In a small pitcher, whisk together the first eight ingredients until smooth and well combined. You can also play with the measurements to adjust to your taste.

2. Transfer to a blender, add the Cool Whip, coffee creamer, and ice then blend. When you no longer hear the ice being crushed, it's ready!

3. Divide equally into two mason jars. Insert straws and enjoy!

Beverages

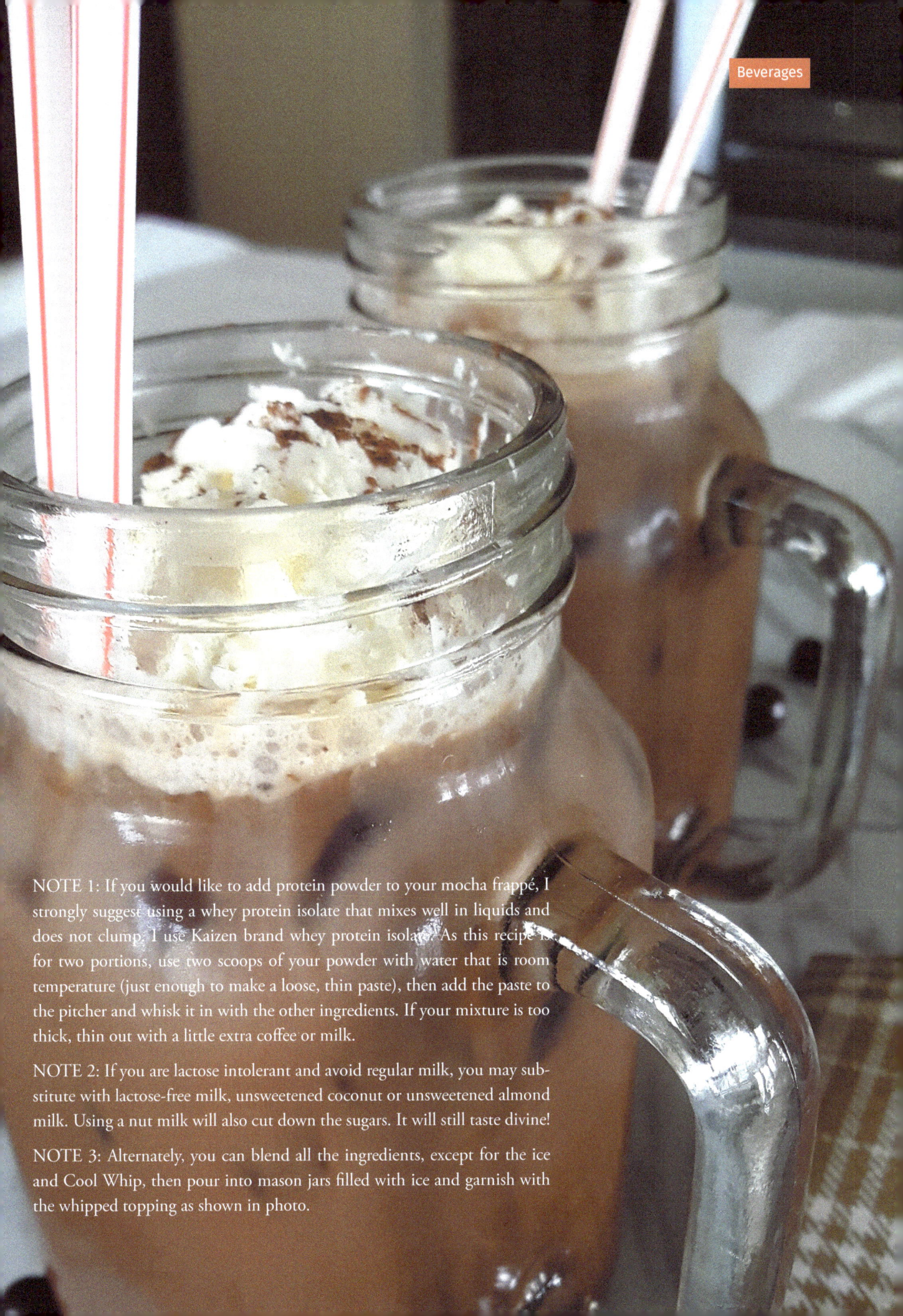

NOTE 1: If you would like to add protein powder to your mocha frappé, I strongly suggest using a whey protein isolate that mixes well in liquids and does not clump. I use Kaizen brand whey protein isolate. As this recipe is for two portions, use two scoops of your powder with water that is room temperature (just enough to make a loose, thin paste), then add the paste to the pitcher and whisk it in with the other ingredients. If your mixture is too thick, thin out with a little extra coffee or milk.

NOTE 2: If you are lactose intolerant and avoid regular milk, you may substitute with lactose-free milk, unsweetened coconut or unsweetened almond milk. Using a nut milk will also cut down the sugars. It will still taste divine!

NOTE 3: Alternately, you can blend all the ingredients, except for the ice and Cool Whip, then pour into mason jars filled with ice and garnish with the whipped topping as shown in photo.

COMFORT COOKING
for Bariatric Post-Ops and Everyone Else!

SUGAR-FREE HOLIDAY EGGNOG!

This is a Christmas miracle! It looks and tastes just like the eggnog you buy in the cartons. There are so many kinds of eggnogs out there but you cannot find any sugar-free ones. Here it is!

INGREDIENTS

One 1-oz. pack sugar-free vanilla instant pudding mix (I use Jell-O brand)

6 c. low fat milk (do not use a nut milk as the pudding mix will not thicken)

2 t. rum extract

1 t. vanilla extract

1 T. Truvia Brown Sugar Blend

½ t. ground cinnamon

¼ t. ground cloves

¼ t. fresh or ground nutmeg

Pinch of salt

INSTRUCTIONS

1. Put pudding mix powder in a large mixing bowl. Whisk in the milk one cup at a time until smooth.
2. Add extracts and spices and blend well. Cover with plastic wrap and chill in the fridge overnight to allow for flavours to blend. If the mixture is too thick, you can add a bit more milk to thin it out.
3. Serve chilled.

NOTE A: I usually pour my eggnog into an empty milk carton and label it.

To serve: Pour one-half cup servings into glasses. For those who will want the alcohol, add two tablespoons (one ounce) of rum per one-half cup and stir well. Add a dollop of sugar-free whipped cream or regular Cool Whip and a dusting of nutmeg.

NOTE B: If you cannot drink dairy, you may substitute milk for unsweetened almond milk. It will not thicken but it will taste wonderful!

Beverages

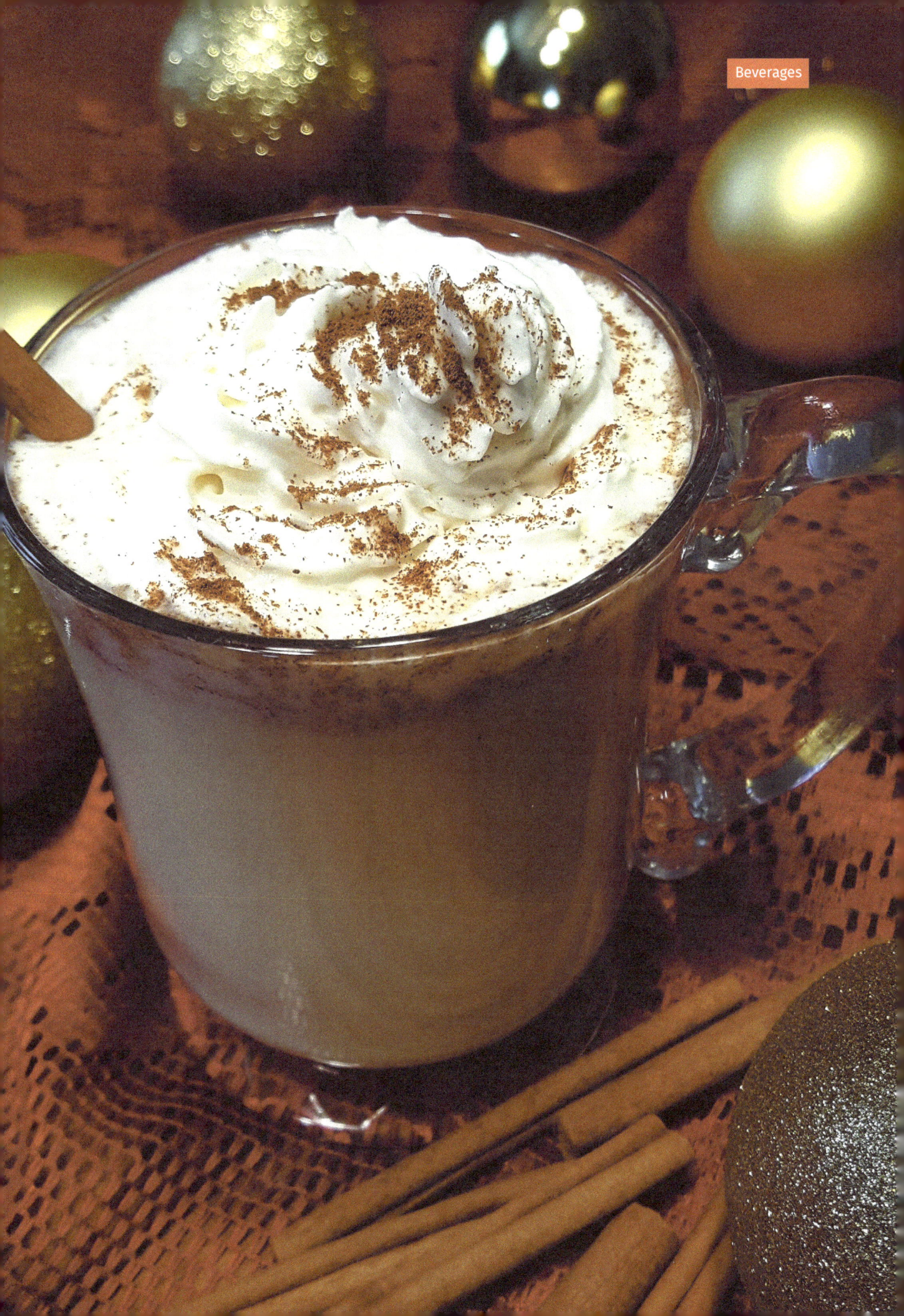

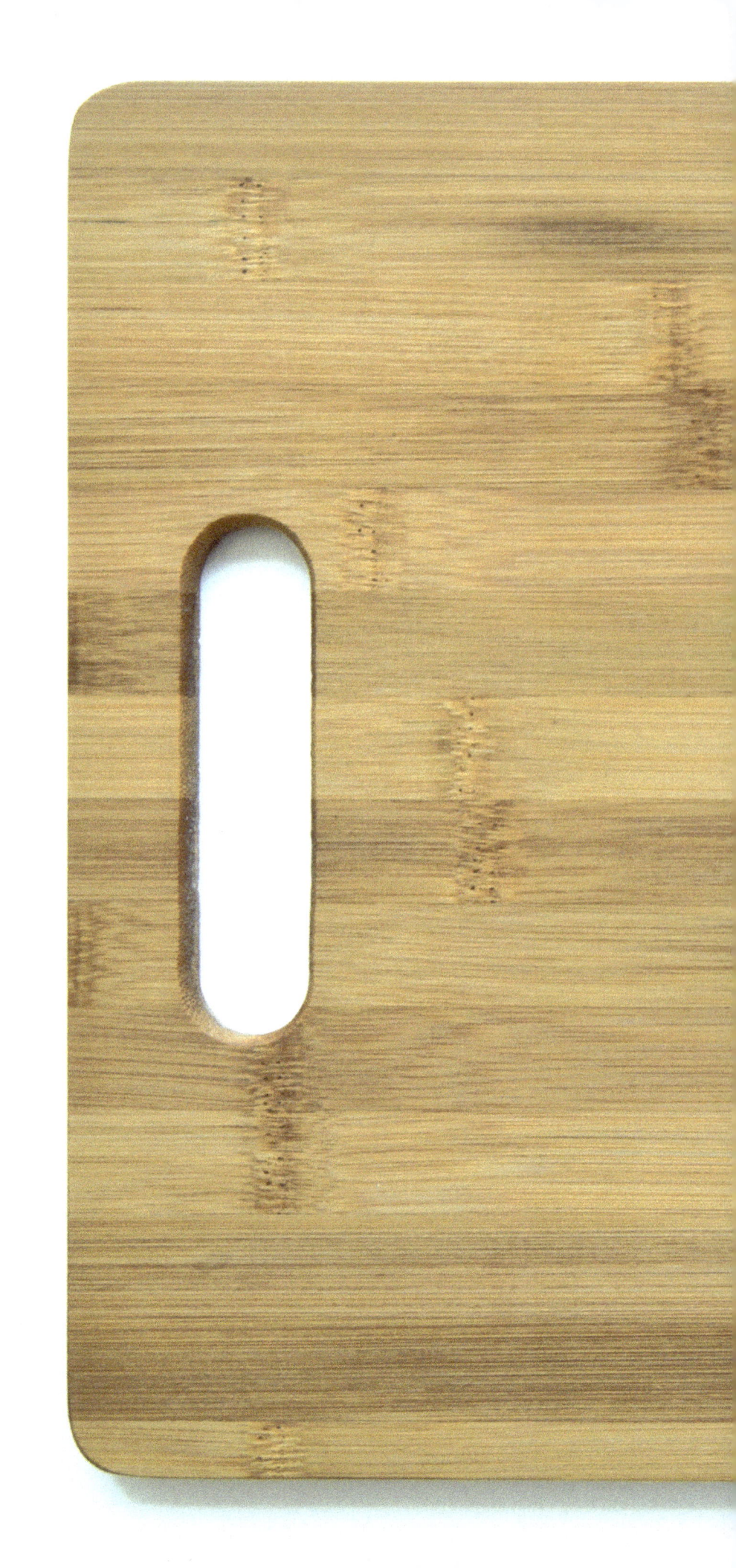

SOUPS AND SALADS

Taco Soup.................................50

Pumpkin Soup............................52

Broccoli Cheese Soup 54

Hearty Beef and Vegetable Soup............56

Comforting Chicken "Noodle" Soup 58

Better Than Canned Tomato Soup...........60

Cobb Salad................................62

Coleslaw..................................64

Taco Salad 66

Caesar Salad 68

TACO SOUP

Love, love, love this soup. I usually make this at least every other week and I freeze the leftovers in one-bowl portions.

INGREDIENTS

1 t. olive oil

1 medium onion, diced

3 garlic cloves, minced

1 red pepper, diced

1 lb. lean ground beef or shredded chicken

1 10-oz. jar salsa

1 large can diced tomatoes

1 packet taco seasoning mix

1 can pinto beans

½ can kidney beans (freeze the rest for another time)

½ can black beans (freeze the rest for another time)

1 handful of frozen mixed vegetables

1 container low-sodium chicken broth

2 T. lime juice

INSTRUCTIONS

1. Heat the olive oil in a soup pot and sauté the onion, garlic, and red pepper until softened and browned.
2. Add the ground meat and cook until nicely browned.
3. Add the salsa, tomatoes, seasoning, beans, and vegetables. (Feel free to add other seasonings if you like, such as more chili powder, garlic powder, oregano, etc.)
4. Add the chicken broth to cover. Bring to a boil then reduce heat. Simmer for 15 to 20 minutes. Add lime and serve!
5. I like to give a shake of hot sauce and fresh ground black pepper to my bowl.

NOTE A: If using shredded chicken, add it to the pot during the last 10 minutes of simmering.

NOTE B: Rules for eating soup are liquid first, then the chunks.

Soups And Salads

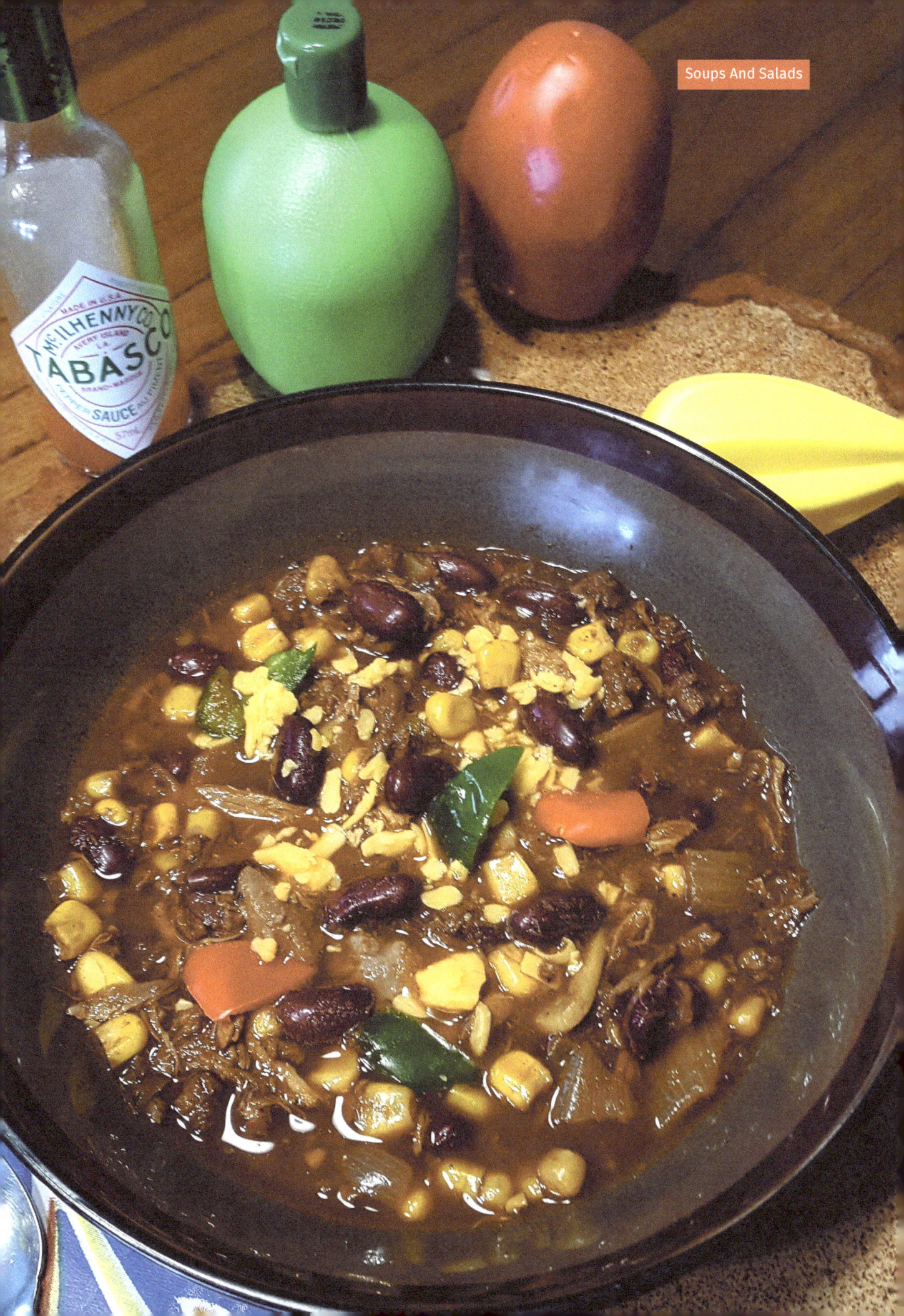

PUMPKIN SOUP

I cannot say enough about this soup. It has become our favourite any time of the year, and it is so special that I frequently serve it to guests when I have a dinner party.

INGREDIENTS

- 1 T. butter
- 1 medium onion, chopped
- 3 cloves garlic, chopped
- 1 T. curry powder
- 1 t. ground cumin
- 1 t. thyme
- ¼ t. cayenne pepper
- ½ t. paprika
- 1 t. ground ginger
- ¼ t. nutmeg
- 1 T. chicken broth soup mix powder (I use Knorr)
- ½ c. peanut butter
- One 15-oz. can pumpkin puree (not pie filling)
- 1 Granny Smith apple, chopped
- 4 c. low-sodium chicken broth
- 1 t. hot sauce (I use Sriracha)
- Ground black pepper
- Seasoned salt

INSTRUCTIONS

1. Gather together your spices, measure, and place in a small bowl. Measure the curry powder separately. Set aside.
2. In a soup pot, sauté the onions and garlic in the butter over medium–low heat until slightly softened. Add the curry powder and cook for one minute.
3. Add the peanut butter, pumpkin, apple, spices, and chicken broth. Combine well and bring to a boil.
4. Reduce heat to very low so it barely boils. Cover and simmer for 15 minutes. Stir occasionally.
5. Remove from heat and let cool. When cooled enough to use an immersion blender, puree until smooth.
6. Adjust salt and pepper to your taste. I find that seasoned salt adds extra flavour. Ladle into bowls and enjoy this unique flavoured soup!

NOTE: For those who would like, you can add a scoop of unflavoured whey protein isolate powder (one that mixes smoothly in liquid), to up the protein in this soup. First, dissolve the powder in a small amount of water until you have a smooth paste, then mix it well into your hot bowl of soup.

Soups And Salads

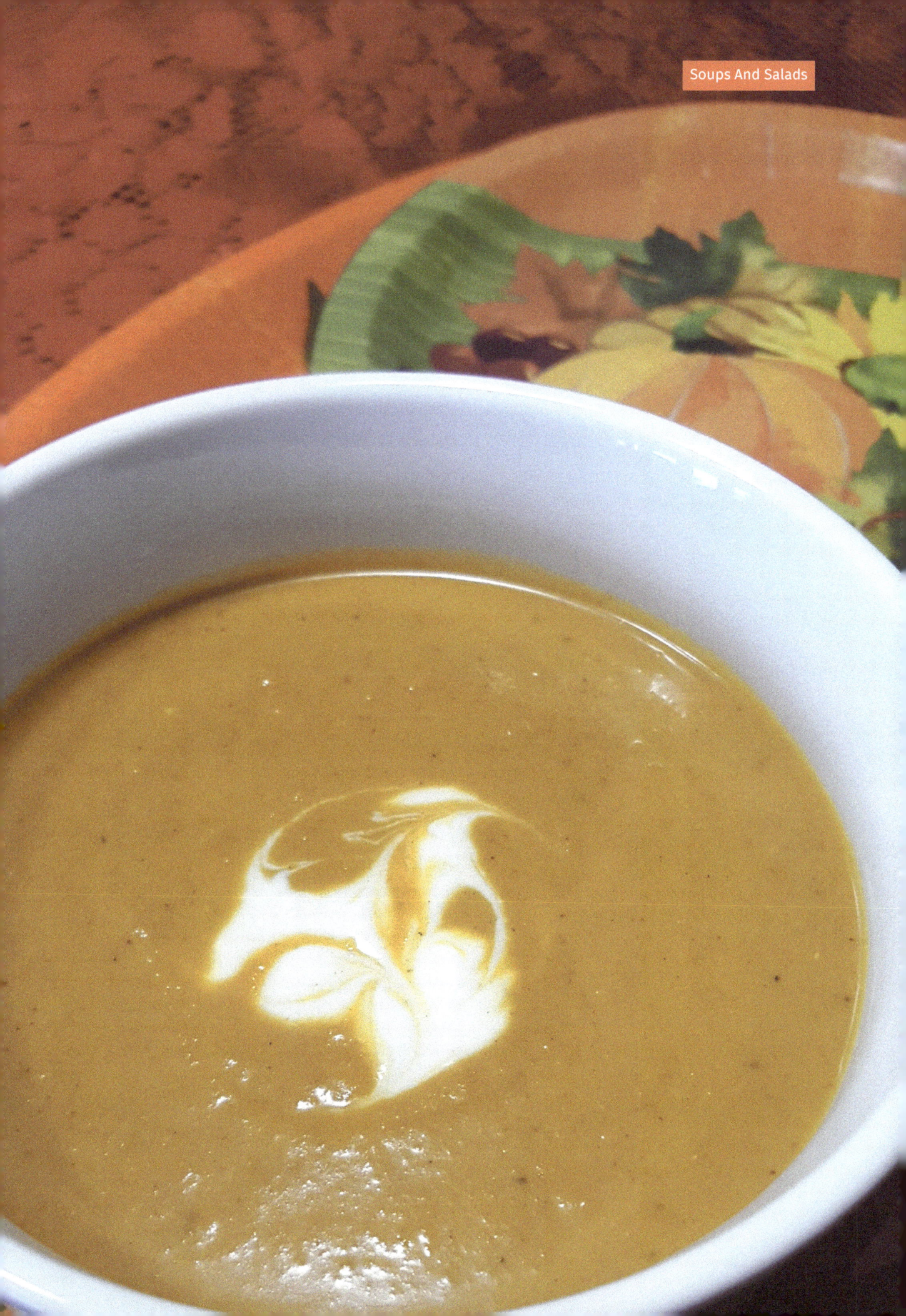

BROCCOLI CHEESE SOUP

Another one of my favourite soups. Cheesy and rich without loads of fat, this is true comfort in a bowl.

INGREDIENTS

- 2 T. salted butter
- 2 cloves garlic, minced
- 1 onion, finely chopped
- 16 oz. fresh broccoli, chopped
- 1 box (900 mL) low-sodium chicken broth
- 1 c. reduced-fat cheddar cheese, shredded
- 1 c. low-fat milk
- 1 c. unsweetened almond milk
- 1 T. garlic powder
- 1 packet chicken bouillon
- 1 T. yellow mustard
- ½ t. black pepper
- ½ t. sea salt
- 1/8 t. cayenne pepper
- 1 t. cheddar cheese popcorn seasoning
- ¼ c. cornstarch
- 1 c. water
- 1 shake liquid smoke (optional but good!)

INSTRUCTIONS

1. In a soup pot, melt butter over medium–low heat. Add onion and garlic and cook until softened.
2. Add the broccoli and the chicken broth and simmer on low until broccoli is tender (about 10 to 15 minutes).
3. Reduce heat to low and stir in cheese until melted. Mix in both milks, garlic powder, chicken bouillon, mustard, and other seasonings. Combine well.
4. In a small bowl, stir cornstarch into water to dissolve. Add to soup and bring up to a boil. Cook uncovered until thickened (about three minutes) stirring frequently.
5. Add a shake of liquid smoke.
6. To serve, ladle into bowls and finish it off with some freshly ground pepper!

NOTE: You may add protein powder to this soup as well. See Pumpkin Soup note for details.

Soups And Salads

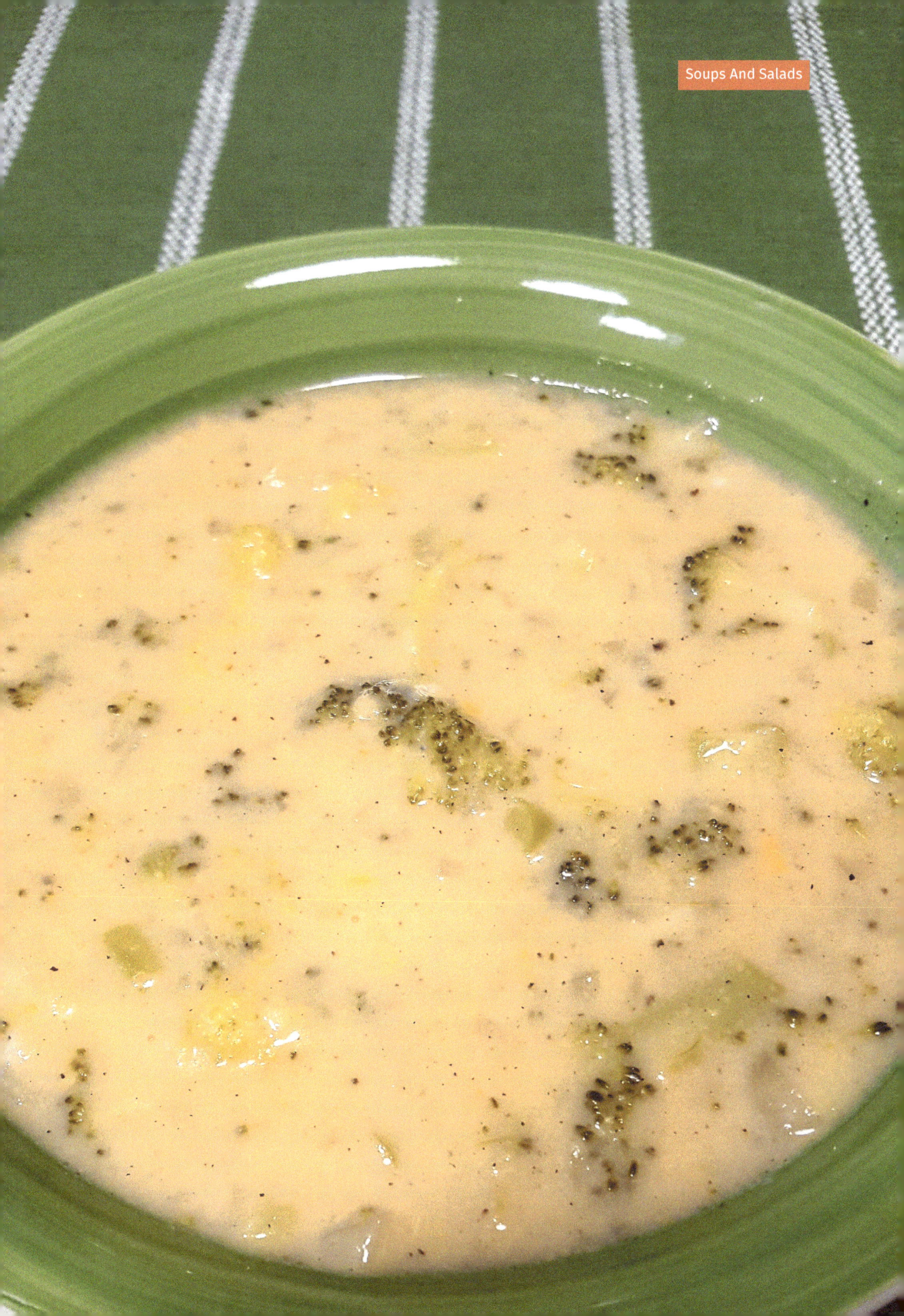

COMFORT COOKING
for Bariatric Post-Ops and Everyone Else!

HEARTY BEEF AND VEGETABLE SOUP

If you haven't guessed it by now, all my soups are my favourite. One is no better than the other. I just know that whenever I feel like soup, I have wonderful choices and I will never be disappointed. Love beef and veggies in this great tasting and satisfying soup!

INGREDIENTS

½ lb. lean ground beef

½ T. olive oil

½ T. butter

2 cloves garlic, minced

1 medium onion, diced

1 large carrot, sliced thin

1 stalk celery, thinly sliced

⅓ c. frozen peas

4 oz. white sweet potato, cut into cubes

½ c. cut frozen green beans

1 container low-sodium beef broth (about 5 c.)

2 packets beef bouillon (I use Knorr OXO)

5 c. water

⅓ c. tomato paste

2 T. no-sugar-added ketchup (I use Heinz)

1 t. seasoned salt

½ t. ground pepper

½ t. garlic powder

½ t. thyme

1 t. onion powder

1 t. dried parsley

1 t. granular sweetener (I use Stevia In The Raw granular)

Pinch of cayenne pepper

1 t. dill weed

1 shake liquid smoke

1 T. cornstarch mixed with a little water

INSTRUCTIONS

1. In a soup pot, melt olive oil and butter over medium–low heat. Add onions and garlic. Cook until softened, then add ground beef and cook until browned.

2. Add all the vegetables, liquids, bouillon, tomato paste, ketchup, seasonings, and liquid smoke. Simmer on low for 45 minutes until vegetables are soft.

3. Add the cornstarch mixture and boil for an additional two minutes.

4. Adjust salt and pepper to your taste.

5. Enjoy!

NOTE: Rules for eating soup are liquid first, then the chunks.

Soups And Salads

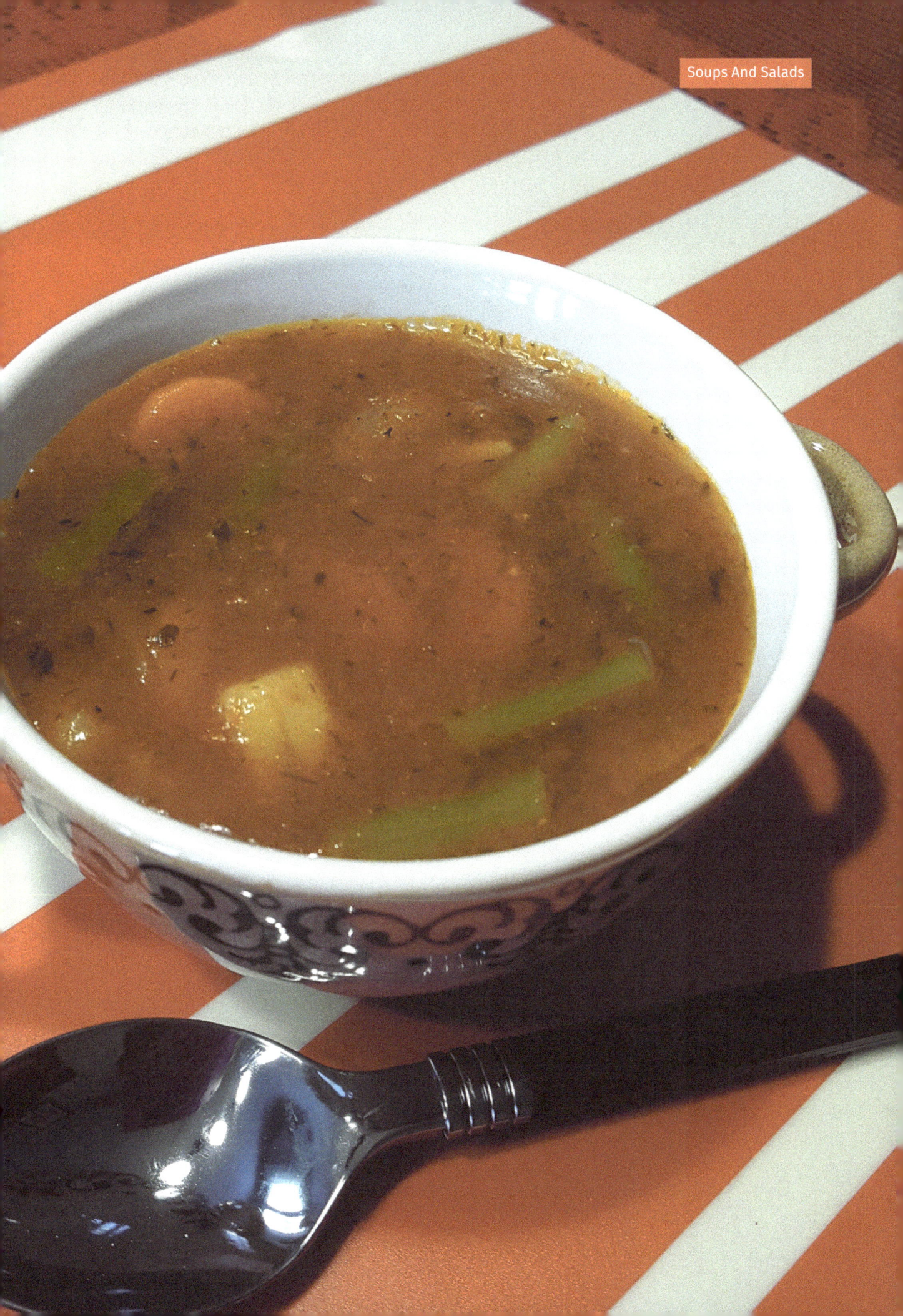

COMFORT COOKING
for Bariatric Post-Ops and Everyone Else!

COMFORTING CHICKEN "NOODLE" SOUP

This one feels like a hug from Mom. It's the ultimate comfort in a bowl. Add a few crêpe "noodles" and enjoy. Even better, when you have a bad cold! Save prep time and buy a grocery store rotisserie chicken. Always soft and tender.

INGREDIENTS

- 1 T. olive oil
- 1 chopped onion
- 2 stalks celery, thinly sliced
- 2 carrots, thinly sliced
- 1 T. ginger root, minced
- 4 cloves garlic, minced
- 1 t. sea salt
- ¼ t. black pepper
- ½ t. garlic powder

- 1½ T. chicken soup dry mix (I use Knorr)
- 2 bay leaves
- 1 t. dried parsley
- 2 boneless skinless chicken thighs
- 1 c. chopped rotisserie chicken, skin removed
- 1 container low-sodium chicken broth
- 5 c. water
- 1 Low-Carb Crêpe, cut into noodle form (recipe found in Sides)

INSTRUCTIONS

1. Place olive oil in a large soup pot and add onion. Sauté on medium heat till glossy. Add chopped garlic and ginger and continue to sauté for a few minutes more.
2. Add carrots, celery, salt, pepper, garlic powder, and dry chicken soup mix. Combine well.
3. Add chicken broth, water, chicken thighs, bay leaves, and parsley. Cover and simmer on low for 30 minutes.
4. Remove chicken thighs and shred. Return the meat back to the pot. Simmer on low until vegetables are tender.
5. Remove bay leaves and add rotisserie chicken. Stir the pot a few times. Adjust salt and pepper to your liking.
6. Place cut "noodles" into a bowl and ladle the hot soup overtop. Enjoy!

NOTE: One Low-Carb Crêpe yields enough "noodles" for four servings. Rules for eating soup are liquid first, then the chunks.

Soups And Salads

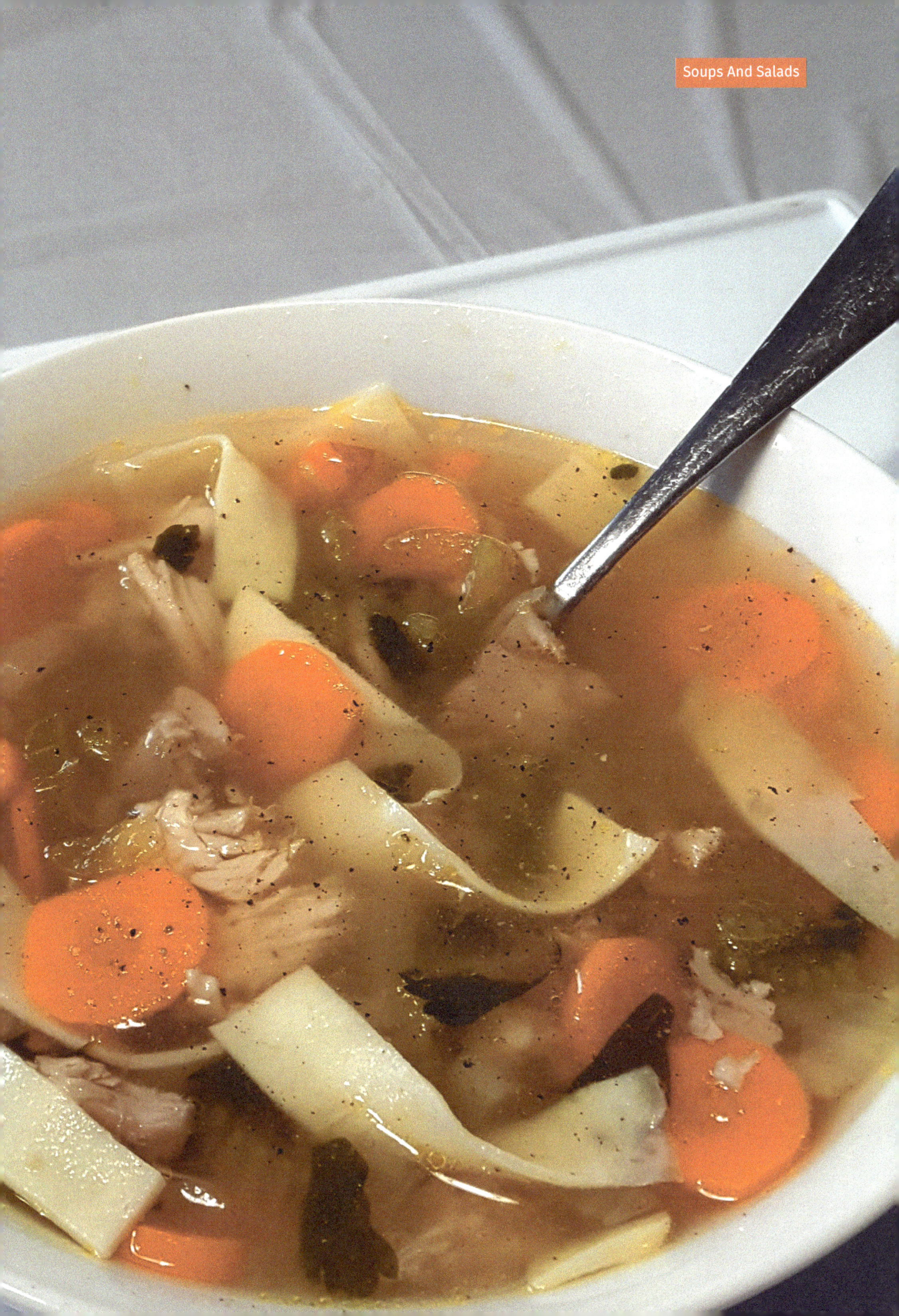

BETTER THAN CANNED TOMATO SOUP

How does one resist a bowl of an old-time childhood favourite? You don't. You pair it with a grilled cheese sandwich using the Low-Carb Flatbread recipe in this book.

INGREDIENTS

Serves four to five

- 1½ small cans (156 mL can) tomato paste
- 5 c. low-sodium chicken or vegetable broth
- ½ c. 1% milk
- ¼ c. unsweetened almond milk
- 1 t. sea salt
- ½ t. black pepper
- 1 t. garlic powder
- 1 t. onion powder
- ½ t. dried Italian seasoning
- 1 T. parmesan cheese
- 3 T. plus 1 t. Truvia Baking Blend
- 1 t. cheddar cheese flavoured popcorn seasoning
- 1 t. ketchup-flavoured popcorn seasoning
- 1 T. butter

INSTRUCTIONS

1. Place all the ingredients into a large soup pot. Stir till combined.
2. Over medium heat, stirring frequently, warm up slowly and when it starts to boil, turn heat to low.
3. Cook for 10 minutes, making sure it is barely boiling.
4. Adjust salt and pepper to your liking.
5. If soup is too thick, add water or broth. Serve hot with a flatbread cheese sandwich.

NOTE: You may add protein powder to this soup as well. See Pumpkin Soup note for details.

Soups And Salads

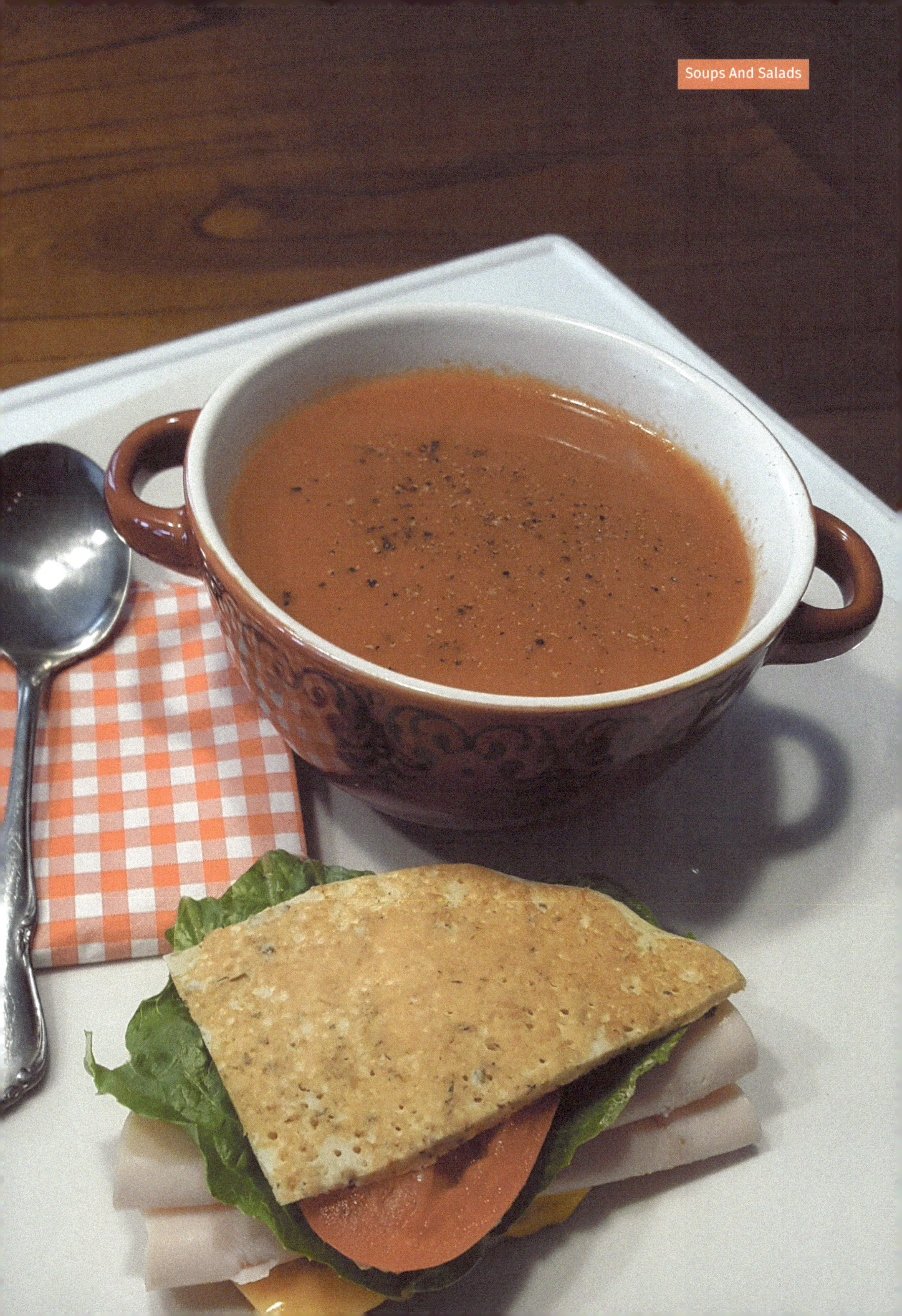

COBB SALAD

This has become my new favourite salad at home or at any restaurant. I love everything in it. It's very filling and full of wonderful protein. This is a winner and will become your new favourite, too!

INGREDIENTS

Serves two

- ½ c. tomatoes, chopped
- 1 c. diced rotisserie chicken
- ½ c. cucumber, chopped
- ¼ c. walnuts or pecans
- 3 c. romaine lettuce, chopped
- 1 hard-cooked egg, halved
- ½ c. blue cheese, crumbled
- ¼ c. bacon, crumbled
- ½ avocado, cubed

DRESSING

- 2 T. olive oil
- 1 T. balsamic vinegar
- 1 T. lemon juice
- 1 t. Dijon mustard
- Few drops Worcestershire
- ¼ t. garlic powder
- ¼ t. salt
- ¼ t. ground pepper
- Pinch granular sweetener
- 1 t. ranch dressing powder (I use Hidden Valley)

INSTRUCTIONS

1. Lay out all the salad ingredients on a large plate as seen in photo.
2. Combine the dressing ingredients in a small bowl and mix well.
3. Drizzle the dressing on top of the salad. Divide the salad into two portions.
4. Enjoy!

Soups And Salads

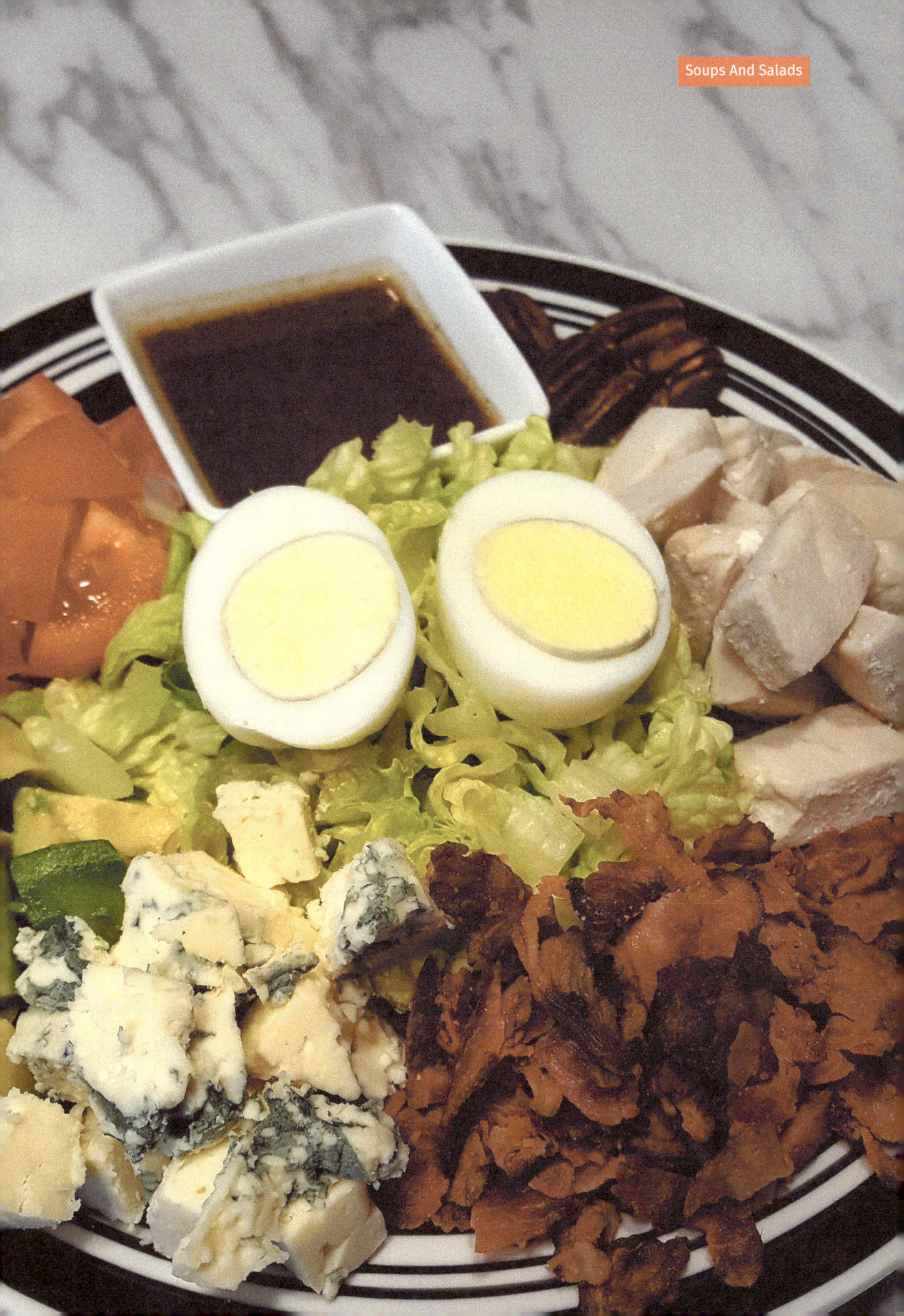

COLESLAW

This is an extraordinary coleslaw recipe that is both crunchy and creamy without adding a lot of fat. It softens up as it sits in the fridge. Enjoy it with any entrée!

INGREDIENTS

4 c. bagged shredded coleslaw

¾ t. salt

2 T. Truvia Baking Blend

2 T. plus 1 t. white vinegar

¼ c. half-fat mayonnaise (I use Hellman's)

¼ c. 0% plain Greek yogurt

Ground black pepper

Unsweetened almond milk to thin out

INSTRUCTIONS

1. Place the coleslaw in a large bowl.
2. In a small bowl, place the remaining ingredients and mix well. Thin the dressing out with a few teaspoons of almond milk, only if necessary.
3. Pour over the coleslaw and mix well making sure to coat evenly.
4. Adjust salt and pepper to taste. Chill before serving.

Soups And Salads

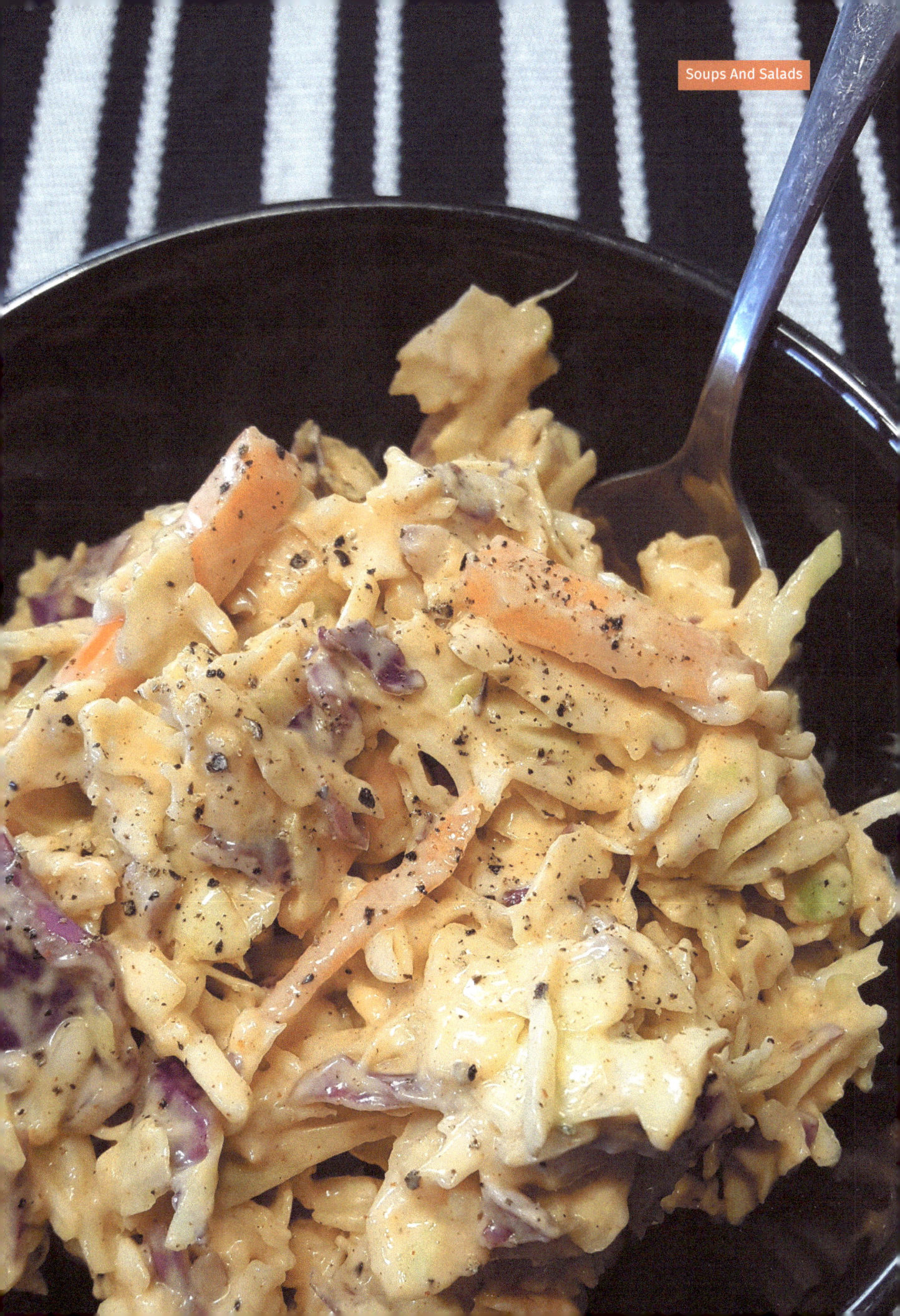

COMFORT COOKING
for Bariatric Post-Ops and Everyone Else!

TACO SALAD

Hang on to your sombreros and prepare for a virtual holiday taste of Mexico all in one bowl! This recipe is flavour-extraordinaire, without all the fat, thanks to thick and creamy Greek yogurt.

INGREDIENTS

Serves about four

- 1 t. olive oil
- 1 lb. lean ground beef
- 1 packet taco seasoning OR your own spice blend
- A few shakes Worcestershire sauce
- Salad fixings: shredded lettuce, grated reduced fat cheddar cheese, chopped tomato, green onion, cubed avocado, etc.

DRESSING

Mix the following ingredients in a small bowl
- ½ c. 0% plain Greek yogurt
- 3–4 t. ranch dressing powder (I use Hidden Valley)
- 2 shakes hot sauce
- ¼ c. no-sugar-added salsa
- ½ t. chili powder

INSTRUCTIONS

1. In a large pan over medium heat, brown the ground beef in olive oil till fully cooked. Add a few shakes of the Worcestershire sauce, then the taco seasoning. Add a little water to thin out if necessary. Blend well, cook for a few minutes longer then set aside.

2. Arrange ground beef and salad fixings in a plate or bowl. Spoon dressing over top and mix.

3. For crunch, crumble a few pork rinds, wisps, cheese crisps, or my Cheese Crackers (recipe found in Appetizers).

Soups And Salads

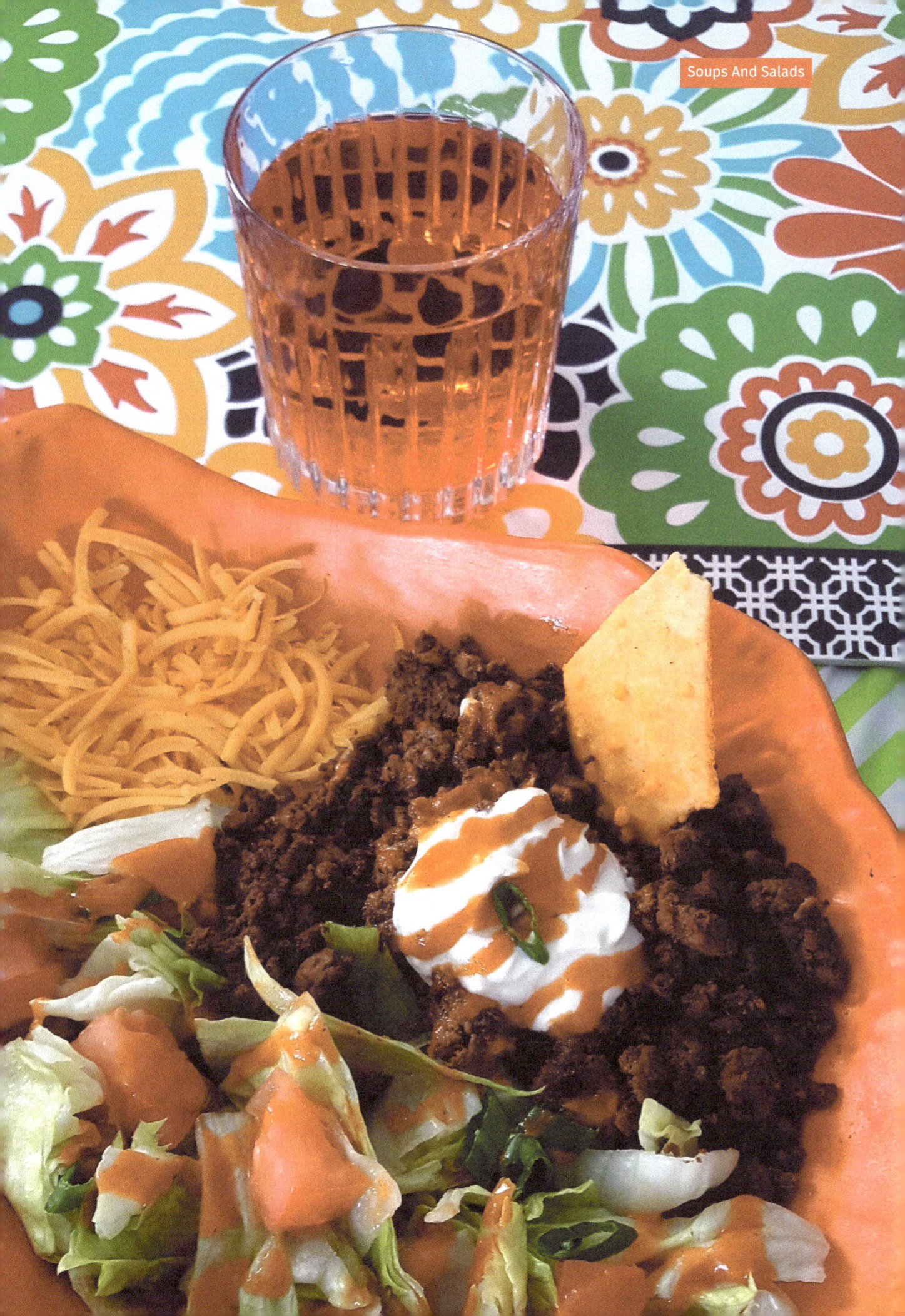

CAESAR SALAD

When I have dinner guests, this is frequently on the menu. It is the easiest salad you can prepare and is always a crowd-pleaser. I also make it for lunches and top it with soft rotisserie chicken for a satisfying meal.

INGREDIENTS

2 bunches Romaine lettuce hearts

¼ c. cooked bacon, crumbled

¼ c. half-fat bottled Caesar salad dressing (I use Renée's)

1 t. lemon juice

1 T. parmesan cheese

Fresh cracked pepper

Handful Cheesy Protein Croutons (recipe found in Appetizers)

INSTRUCTIONS

1. Wash and dry lettuce leaves. Cut into bite-sized pieces and arrange in a salad bowl.
2. Add crumbled bacon and parmesan.
3. In a small bowl, add lemon juice to the Caesar dressing and mix well.
4. Add the dressing to the salad and incorporate to coat. (If need be, you can add another tablespoon of the Caesars dressing.)
5. Add freshly ground pepper. Top with my Cheesy Protein Croutons.

Soups And Salads

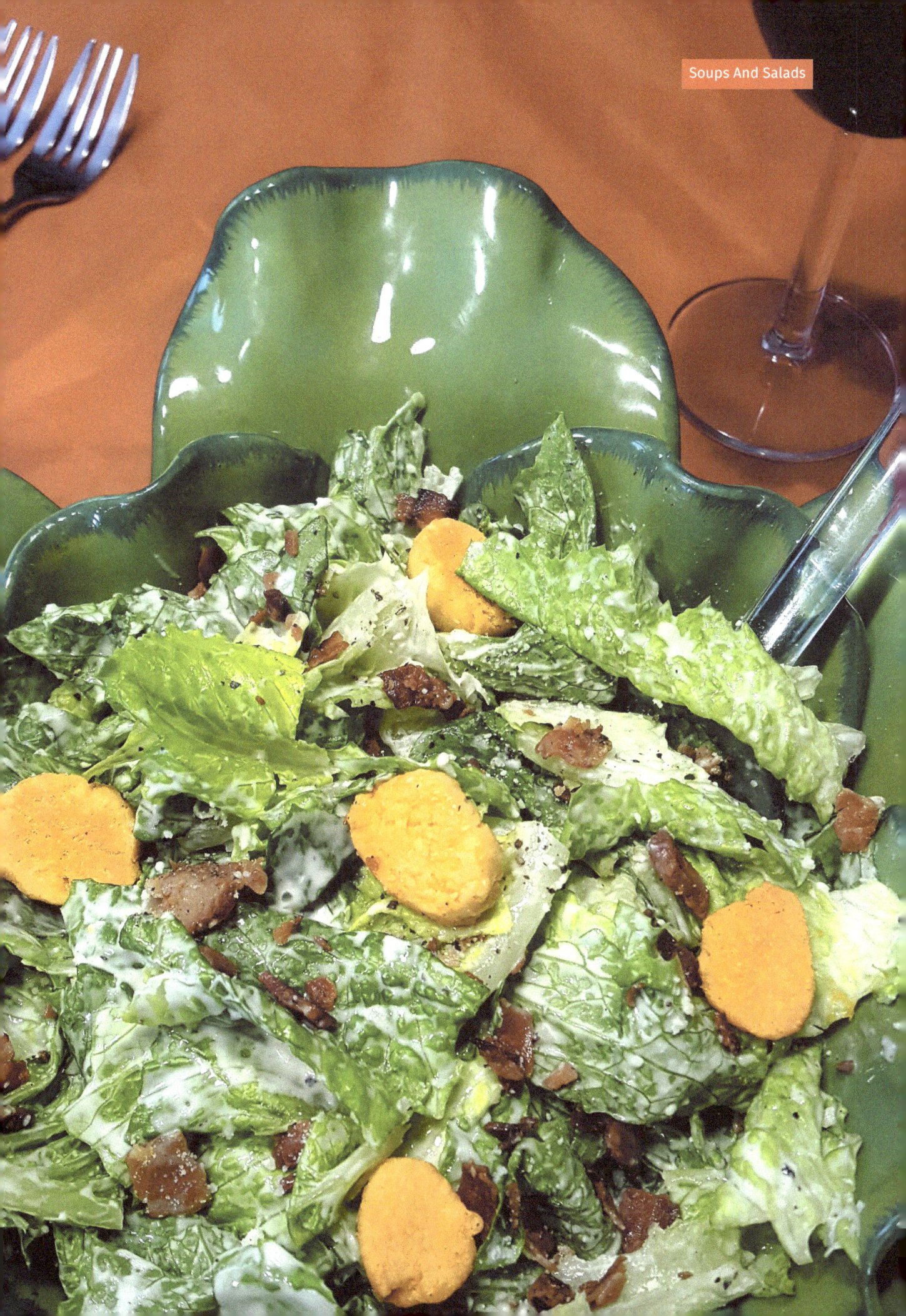

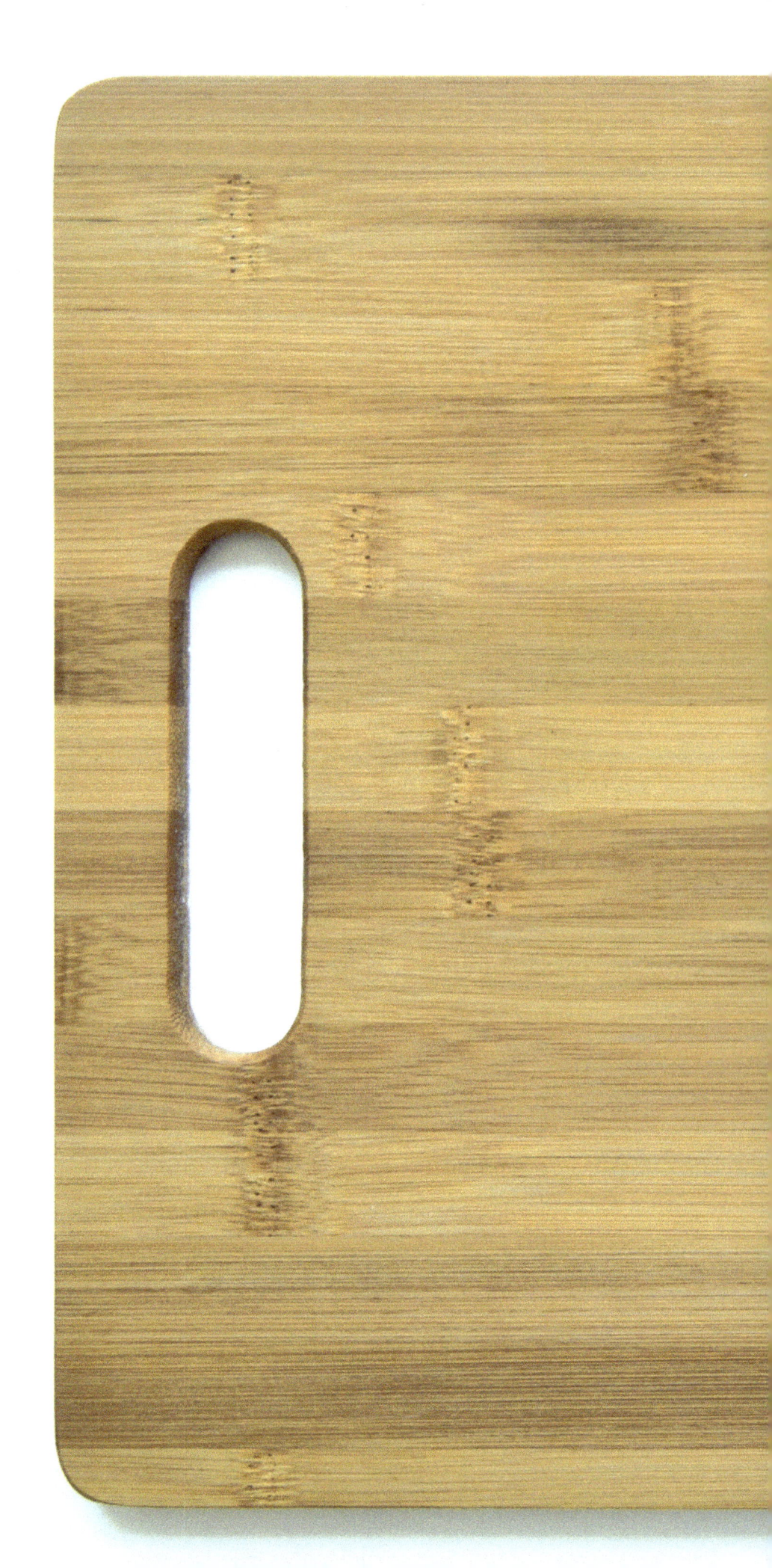

MAIN DISHES

Cheeseburger Pie 72

Chili 74

Shepherd's Pie 76

Beef or Chicken Enchiladas 78

Italian Meatballs 80

Sweet and Sour Meatballs 82

Salisbury Steak 84

Mom's Hungarian Beef Stew 86

Lasagna Skillet 88

Chili Mac Skillet 90

Beef Stroganoff Crêpes 92

Slow Cooker Pulled Pot Roast 94

General Tso's Chicken Makeover 96

Chicken Pot Pie 98

Comfort Chicken Bowl 100

Crispy Chicken Fingers 102

BBQ Ribs 104

Surprise Pizza Crust 106

Pizza! 108

Broiled Cheesy Tuna Casserole 110

Alfredo (Shrimp/Chicken) 112

Egg Foo Yung 114

CHEESEBURGER PIE

This should be one of the first recipes to try. It's soft and tender and will be a family favourite for many years to come. Does it taste like a cheeseburger? Why, yes, it does and it's easy as pie!

INGREDIENTS

- 1¼ lb. lean ground beef
- 1 T. olive oil
- 1 medium onion, diced
- Salt and ground pepper to taste
- ¼ c. no-sugar-added ketchup (I use Heinz)
- 1 T. yellow mustard
- ⅓ c. original baking mix (such as Bisquick)
- 1 c. 1% milk
- 2 eggs
- 4 oz. reduced-fat cheddar cheese, shredded
- Toppings: ketchup, mustard, onions, pickle slices

INSTRUCTIONS

Pre-heat oven to 400°F.

1. Spray a 9-inch pie plate with cooking spray.
2. Sauté onions in olive oil over medium–low heat until tender. Add the ground beef and brown for about six minutes, stirring frequently until fully cooked. Drain excess liquid from the pan, then add salt, pepper, mustard, and ketchup. Set aside.
3. In a medium-sized bowl, combine Bisquick, milk, and eggs until well blended. Stir in cheese.
4. Spoon ground beef into prepared pie plate, then carefully pour the Bisquick mixture over the ground beef. Bake for 25 to 30 minutes or until knife in centre comes out clean.
5. Cut into wedges and serve with burger toppings. Enjoy!

Main Dishes

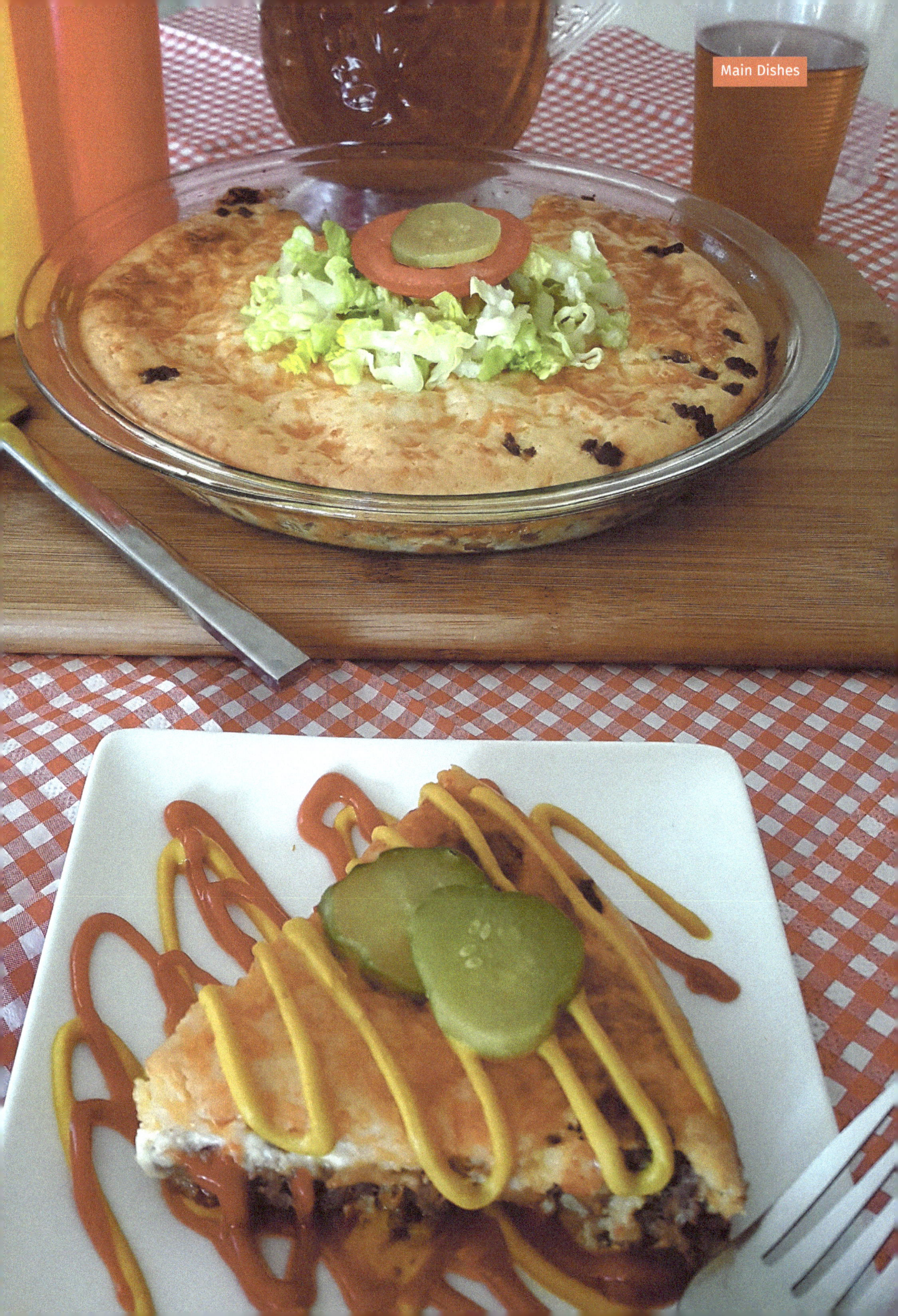

COMFORT COOKING
for Bariatric Post-Ops and Everyone Else!

CHILI

One of the best chili recipes ever! It may seem like a lot of ingredients but, believe me, the result is well worth it! I make sure to have this chili in single portions stored in the freezer so I can have it any time. I especially love a bowl for lunch during the winter months when I need to warm up!

INGREDIENTS

- 1½ lb. lean ground beef
- ¼ c. cooked and crumbled bacon
- 1 T. olive oil
- 1 large onion, diced
- 1 green pepper, diced
- 1 small jalapeno pepper, minced
- 4 garlic cloves, minced
- 1½ t. sea salt
- ½ t. ground pepper
- 5 T. chili powder
- 1 t. ground cumin
- 1 t. dried oregano
- ½ t. ground cinnamon
- 1 T. unsweetened cocoa powder
- 1 T. Truvia Brown Sugar Blend
- 1 28-oz. can diced tomatoes
- ½ c. no-sugar salsa
- 1 can of beer, your choice
- 1 can (15 oz.) pinto beans, drained
- ½ can red kidney beans, drained (freeze the other half for another pot!)
- ½ can black beans, drained (freeze the other half for another pot!)
- A small handful of corn for colour
- 3 T. lime juice
- 2 t. yellow mustard
- 2 squirts liquid smoke

INSTRUCTIONS

1. In a soup pot, brown the meat in olive oil over high heat. Add the bacon, onions, peppers, and garlic and cook until softened.
2. Add all the spices and stir as the mixture cooks for a few minutes.
3. Stir in the tomatoes, salsa, beer, beans, and corn.
4. Bring to a boil then lower the heat to a simmer for about 50 minutes.
5. Add the lime juice, mustard, and liquid smoke. Give it a stir and add more salt and pepper, if necessary.
6. If you prefer a looser chili, add one-half cup of low-sodium chicken broth.
7. Serve in bowls garnished with a dollop of 0% plain Greek yogurt, thinly sliced onions and a touch of reduced-fat shredded cheddar.

Main Dishes

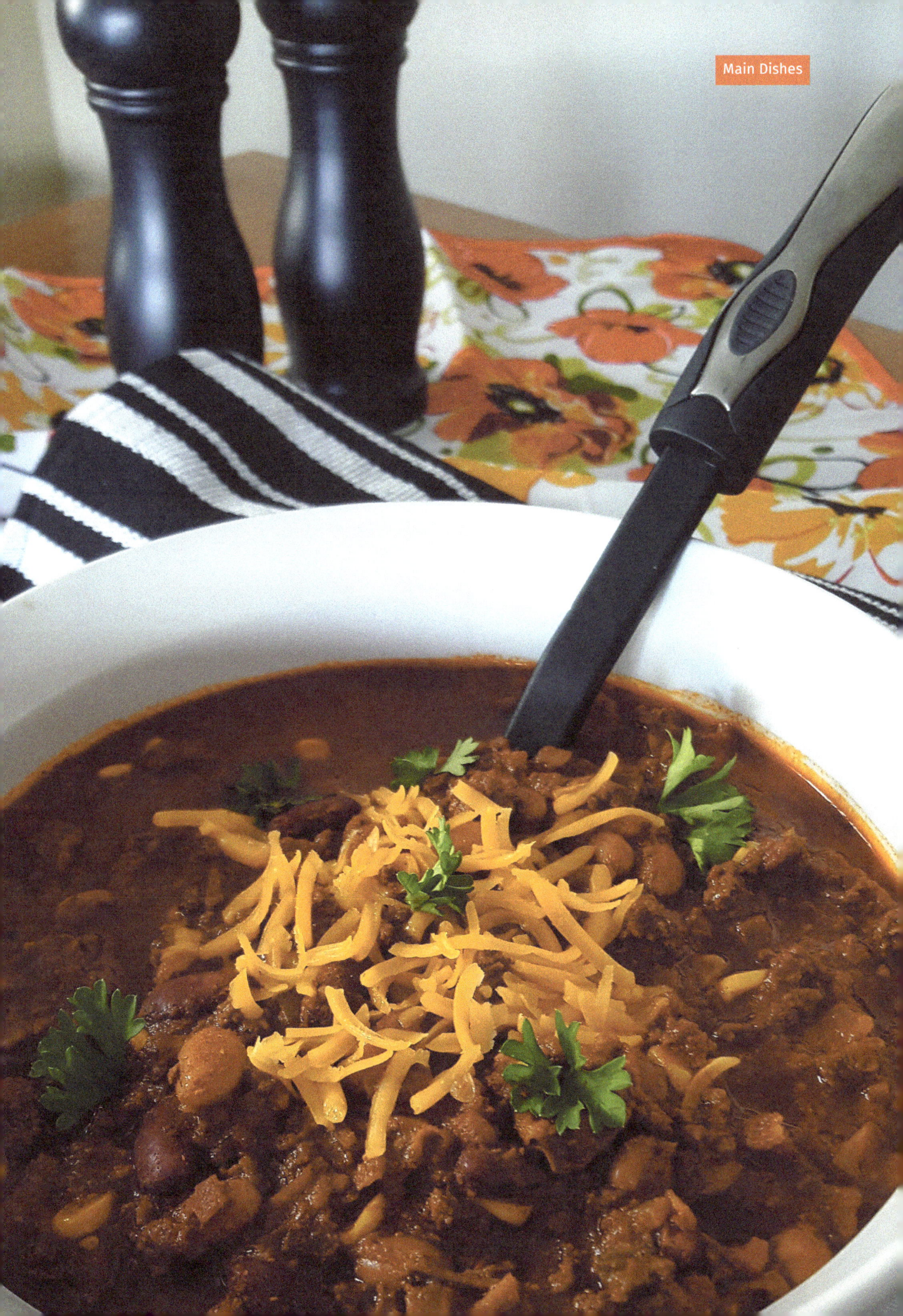

SHEPHERD'S PIE

Another comfort favourite you should never go without. Your family will thank you. Here, the traditional potato topping is replaced with a combination of cauliflower and white flesh sweet potato, mashed to a perfectly silky texture. The result is nothing less than the flavours of your old fave!

INGREDIENTS

- 1 T. olive oil
- 1 lb. lean ground beef
- ½ medium onion, chopped
- 2 cloves garlic, minced
- ½ t. salt
- ¼ t. black pepper
- 1 t. garlic powder
- 1 t. paprika
- ½ t. dried thyme
- 1 packet beef bouillon (I use Knorr)
- 1 T. no-sugar-added ketchup (I use Heinz)
- 1 shake of hot sauce
- 2 T. white flour
- ¾ c. low-sodium beef broth
- 1 T. Worcestershire sauce
- ¼ c. reduced-fat cheddar cheese, shredded
- 1 T. jarred Alfredo sauce
- 1 c. frozen mixed vegetables, boiled to soften

INSTRUCTIONS

1. In a large saucepan, over medium heat, sauté onions and garlic in olive oil until tender.
2. Add ground beef and all spices and brown until fully cooked. Add ketchup and hot sauce and mix well.
3. Sprinkle meat with flour and add beef broth and Worcestershire sauce. Stir until it begins to thicken.
4. Turn down heat to low and add cheese, Alfredo sauce, and vegetables, stirring to combine. Cover and cook on a low simmer for 10 minutes. Set aside. Prepare the "potato" topping.

FAUX MASHED "POTATOES"

- 6 oz. white flesh sweet potato
- 5 large cauliflower florets with stems
- 1 T. butter
- 1 t. onion powder
- ½ t. garlic powder
- ¼ c. reduced fat cheddar cheese
- ½ t. salt
- Ground pepper to taste

Main Dishes

INSTRUCTIONS

1. Boil the cauliflower and white sweet potato in salted water for 12 minutes or until tender. Drain in a colander in the sink and let it steam out for 10 minutes or more to lose as much liquid as possible. Return to pot and add remaining ingredients. Mash till smooth. Taste and adjust salt. (Because you are using sweet potato, you will find that you need a bit more salt.)

Pre-heat oven to 370°F and spray a 9 × 9 glass baking dish with vegetable spray.

2. Add the beef to the baking dish and spoon the potato mixture on top evenly. Spray the top of the potatoes with cooking spray and bake for 25 minutes until browned and bubbly. Broil for 8 to 10 minutes till top browns further. Cool slightly before cutting into squares.

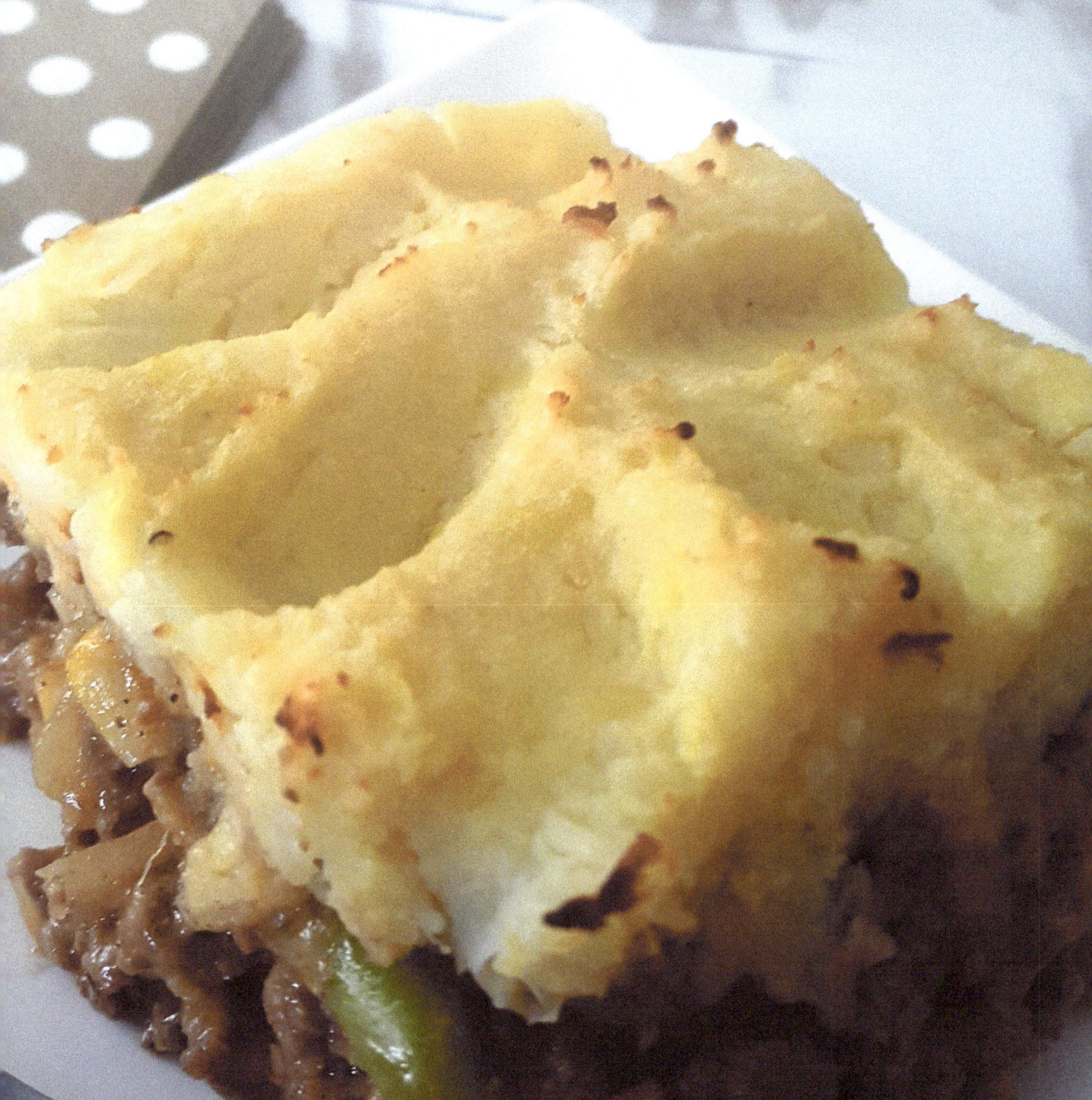

COMFORT COOKING
for Bariatric Post-Ops and Everyone Else!

BEEF OR CHICKEN ENCHILADAS

As you can see, Mexican food is one of my favourites and this one doesn't disappoint. This recipe makes a nice-sized layered casserole that's quite filling and you should have leftovers to freeze.

INGREDIENTS

- 1 lb. lean ground beef or 2 c. rotisserie chicken
- ½ T. olive oil
- 1 medium onion, chopped
- 1 small jalapeno pepper, minced
- 2 garlic cloves, minced
- 1 T. chili powder
- 1 T. unsweetened cocoa powder
- 1 t. oregano
- 1 t. salt
- ½ t. ground black pepper
- 1 t. garlic powder
- ½ t. paprika
- ½ t. Cajun spice blend
- 2 shakes Worcestershire sauce
- 1 shake Tabasco sauce
- ½ c. no-sugar tomato sauce
- 1 t. lime juice
- 1½ c. reduced-fat cheddar cheese (or a combination of cheddar with Monterey or pepper jack)
- 5 Low-Carb Crêpes (recipe found in Sides)

INSTRUCTIONS

1. Gather all your dry spices, measure and place in a plastic bag. Set aside.
2. In a large sauce pan, over medium heat, sauté onions, garlic, and pepper until softened. Add meat and brown, adding the spice mix half way. Continue to brown until fully cooked.
3. Reduce heat to low, then add the tomato sauce, Worcestershire, and lime juices. Combine well and cook for an additional three minutes. Remove from heat and set aside.

ENCHILADA SAUCE

- 3 T. vegetable oil
- 1 T. flour
- ¼ c. chili powder
- 2½ c. low sodium chicken broth
- ⅓ c. tomato paste
- 1 t. oregano
- ½ t. salt and ¼ t. ground black pepper
- 1 t. ground cumin
- ½ t. garlic powder
- 1 t. unsweetened cocoa powder

LISA SHARON BELKIN

Main Dishes

INSTRUCTIONS

1. In a medium-sized pot, heat oil then add flour, smoothing with a wooden spoon. Cook for one minute. Add chili powder and cook for 30 seconds. Add chicken broth, tomato paste, and remaining spices. Stir to combine and bring to a boil.

2. Reduce heat to a simmer and cook for 15 minutes, stirring occasionally. Sauce will begin to thicken. Adjust salt and pepper to taste. Set aside.

TO ASSEMBLE

Pre-heat oven to 350°F and spray an 8 × 8 glass baking dish with vegetable spray.

1. Ladle a bit of sauce onto the bottom of the dish. Place the first crêpe on it. Ladle some meat onto the crêpe, evenly, then a sprinkling of cheese, then some sauce and then the second crêpe. Continue this layering until you are on your fifth crêpe.

2. Top it with the remainder of cheese and bake for 25 to 30 minutes, until bubbly.

3. Remove from oven and cool slightly before cutting into squares.

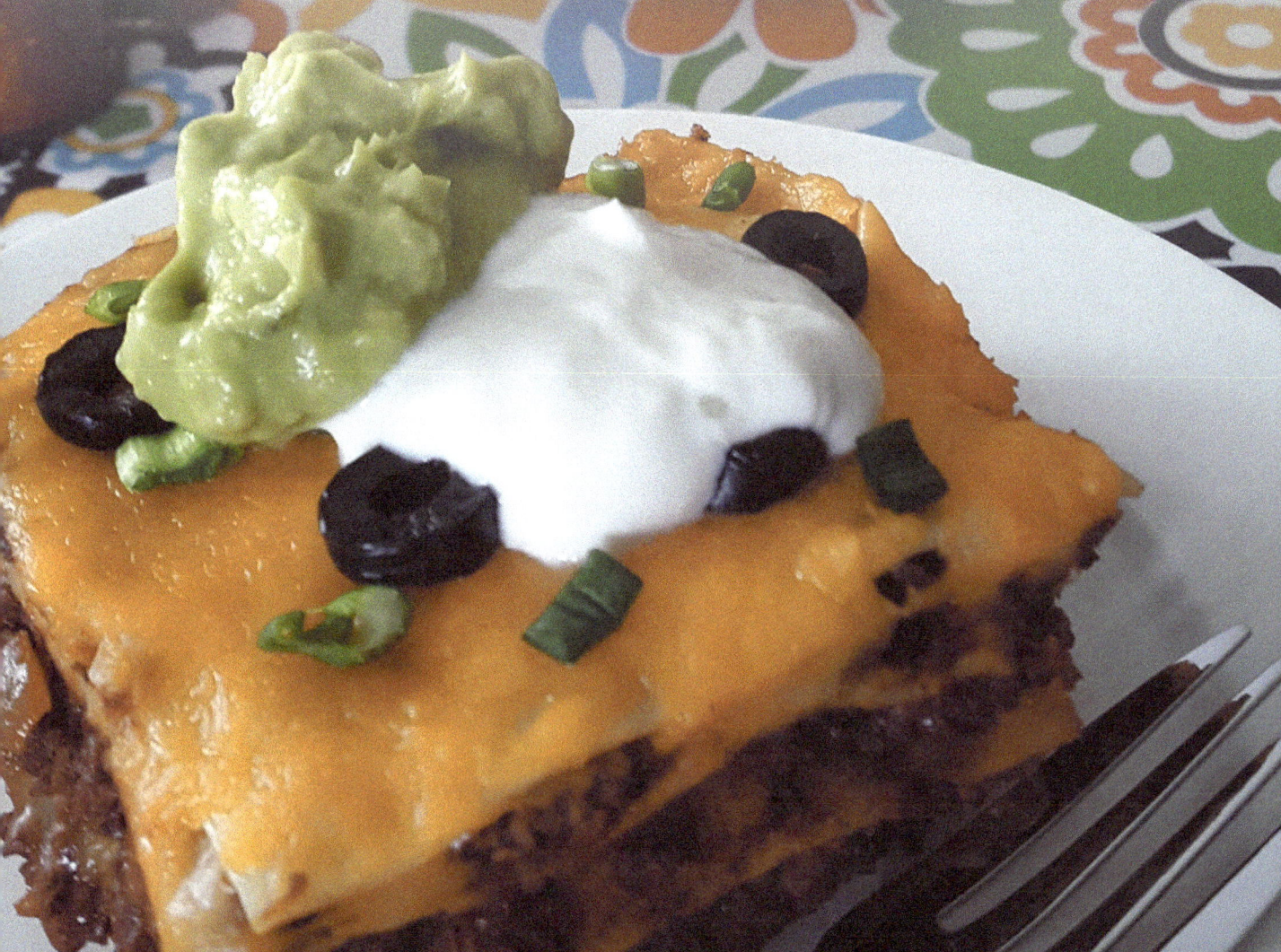

4. Garnish with 0% plain Greek yogurt, sliced green onions, sliced black olives, and guacamole!

ITALIAN MEATBALLS

Mama Mia, these are the best meatballs you will ever make! Soft, easy, and quick to prepare and ever so versatile—eat them from a bowl or overtop some veggie noodles or snuggled inside a Low-Carb Crêpe topped with ricotta and warm marinara sauce.

INGREDIENTS

Makes 16 small or nine large balls

- 1 lb. lean ground beef or mixture of beef and pork
- 1 T. olive oil
- 1 large egg
- ⅓ c. parmesan cheese
- 1 t. salt
- ½ t. ground black pepper
- 3 garlic cloves, minced
- 2 T. dried parsley
- ⅓ c. Italian breadcrumbs mixed into ½ c. water
- 3 c. low-sugar pasta sauce

INSTRUCTIONS

1. In a large bowl, add beef, egg, parmesan, salt, pepper, garlic, parsley, and bread crumb mixture. Combine till well blended.

2. Portion into 16 small or nine large meatballs. I use an ice cream scoop to measure.

3. In a large pot or non-stick skillet, brown the meatballs in olive oil over medium heat, flipping them carefully to brown all sides.

4. Add the sauce and bring to a boil. Then reduce heat to a simmer and cover. Cook for 10 minutes or until fully cooked. Presto!

Main Dishes

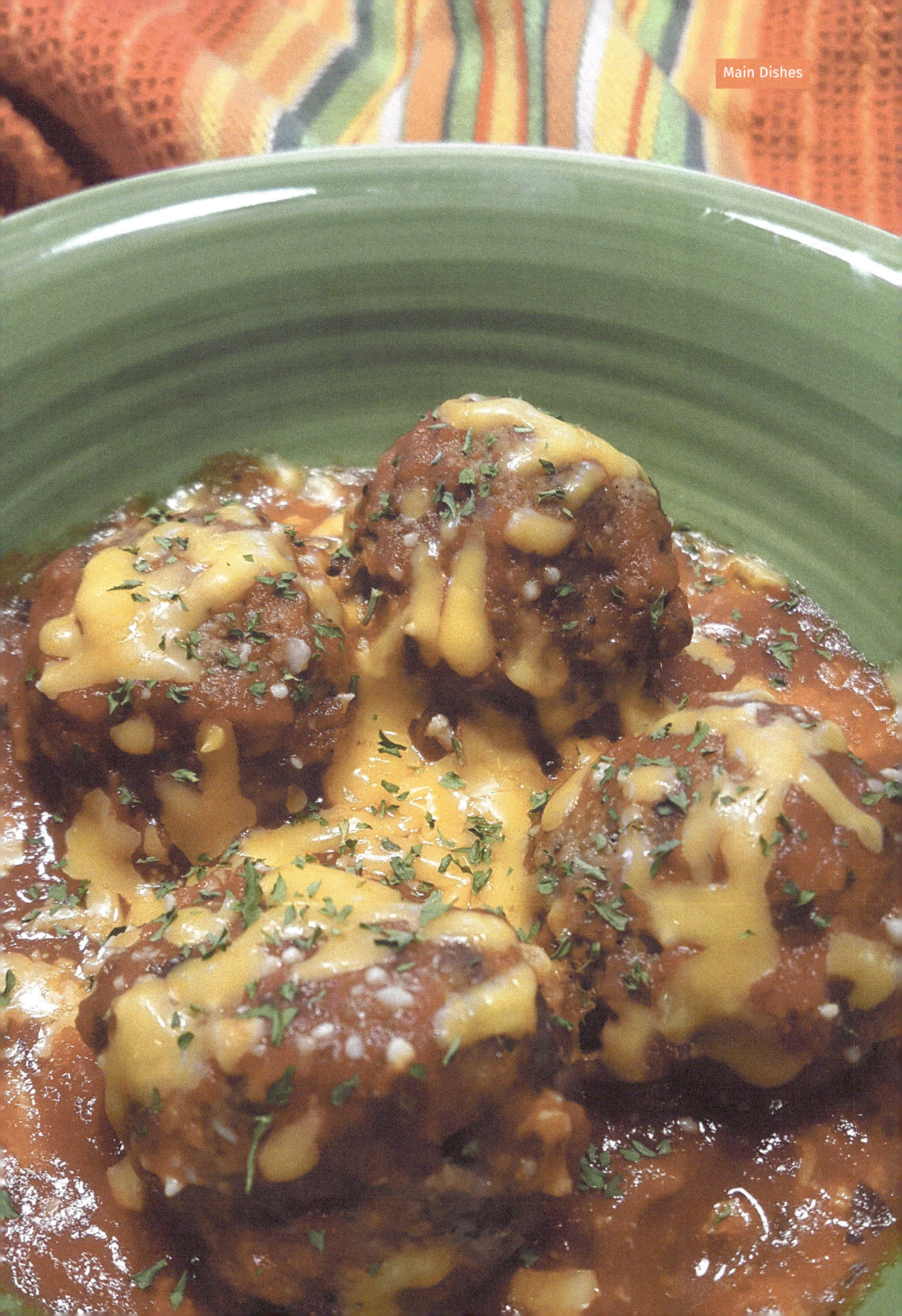

SWEET AND SOUR MEATBALLS

Another versatile dish. Serve in a bowl over Fried "Rice" with Egg Foo Yung, or just on their own! Classic flavour without being a sugar bomb.

INGREDIENTS FOR SWEET AND SOUR SAUCE

- ½ c. water
- ½ c. white vinegar
- ½ c. Truvia Brown Sugar Blend
- 4 t. cornstarch mixed into 1 T. water
- 1 T. soy sauce
- A pinch of salt and pepper

INGREDIENTS FOR MEATBALLS

- 1 lb. lean ground beef
- ½ egg (scramble then measure)
- 1 t. salt
- ½ t. black pepper
- 1½ t. garlic powder
- ¼ c. dry breadcrumbs mixed into less than ¼ c. water
- 1 T. olive oil

INSTRUCTIONS

1. Combine Sauce ingredients in a small pot. Whisk until well blended and simmer over medium–low heat for five minutes, stirring occasionally until thickened. Set aside and make the meatballs.
2. Combine all Meatball ingredients, except for oil, in a large bowl. Mix well.
3. Portion into 16 balls using an ice cream scoop (approximately one and one-half heaping tablespoons of meat per ball).
4. Heat up a non-stick skillet on medium heat with olive oil and brown the meatballs on all sides.
5. Add the Sweet and Sour Sauce and bring up to a boil. Reduce heat to low, cover and simmer for 10 minutes or until fully cooked.
6. Serve as you wish.

Main Dishes

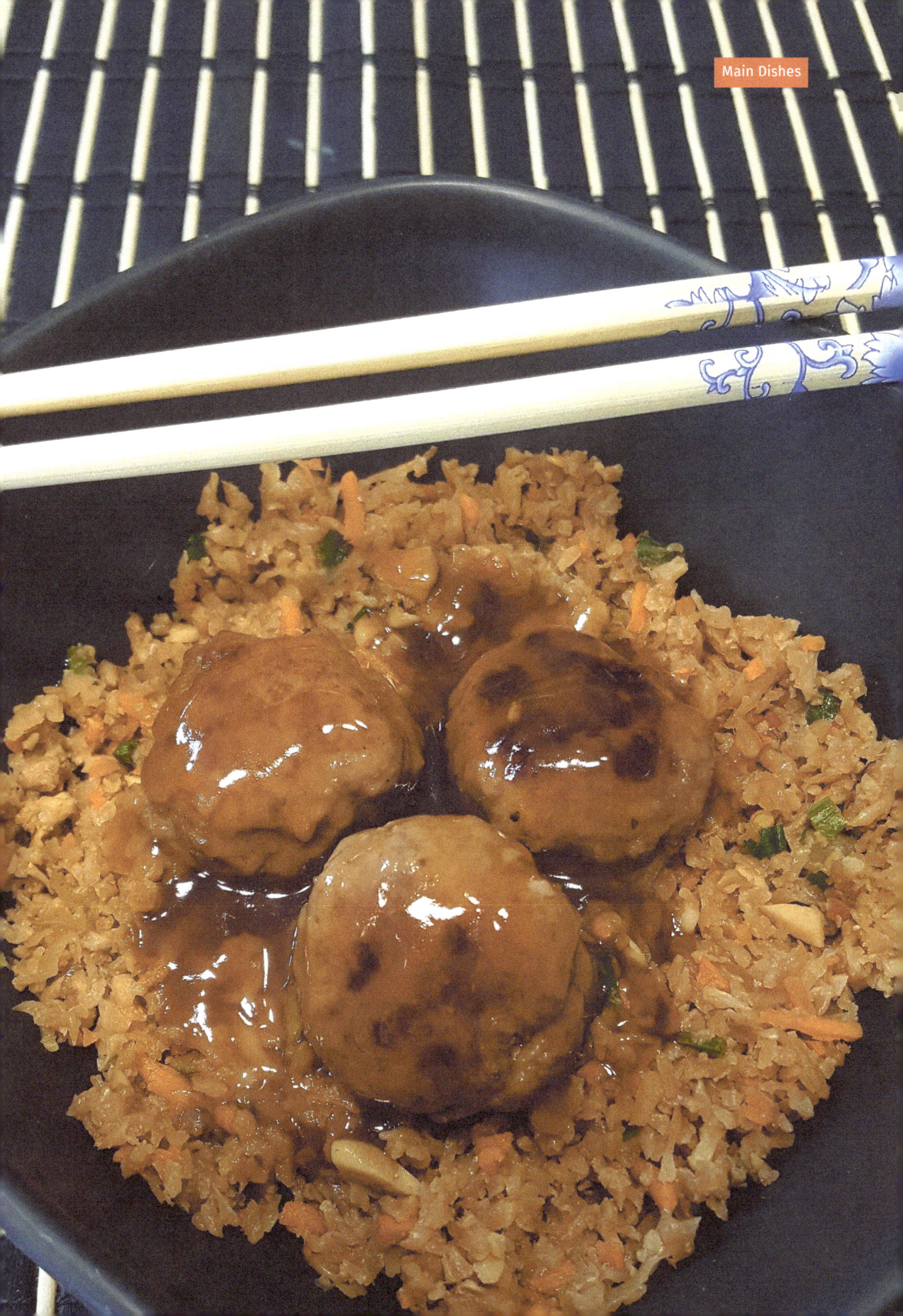

SALISBURY STEAK

An easy comfort classic! Soft and flavourful, with a tangy gravy served over Faux Mashed "Potatoes"! Who wouldn't love a plate like this for dinner?

INGREDIENTS

1 lb. lean ground beef	1 T. cornstarch
1 T. olive oil	2 c. low-sodium beef broth
½ t. black pepper	1 beef bouillon cube or packet (I use OXO)
1 t. salt	3 T. no-sugar-added ketchup (I use Heinz)
½ t. garlic powder	1 T. yellow mustard
1 t. Worcestershire sauce	2 T. parmesan cheese
1 egg	1 t. onion powder
¼ c. plus 1 T. dry bread crumbs	1 shake Worcestershire sauce
1 large onion, sliced	

INSTRUCTIONS

1. Combine the beef, black pepper, salt, garlic powder, Worcestershire sauce, egg, and bread crumbs. Mix well and shape into four equal-sized oval patties.

2. Heat oil in a large skillet over medium heat for about a minute. Place patties in skillet, brown on both sides for about four to five minutes each. Remove from skillet and set aside on a plate.

3. Add the sliced onions to the same skillet, reducing the heat to low and cook for 25 minutes until browned and tender, stirring occasionally. Give the skillet a spray of vegetable spray if necessary.

4. Sprinkle cornstarch over the onions and stir till well combined. Cook for an additional two minutes.

5. Add beef broth and bouillon packet. Raise the heat back up to medium. Add the ketchup, mustard, parmesan, onion powder, and shake of Worcestershire sauce. Stir to combine, then place the patties back in the pan.

6. Cover, reduce heat to a low simmer for about 15 minutes, till flavours combine and sauce is slightly thickened. Remove from heat, uncover, and allow to thicken up a bit more. Serve warm next to some great tasting Faux Mashed "Potatoes." Yummy!

Main Dishes

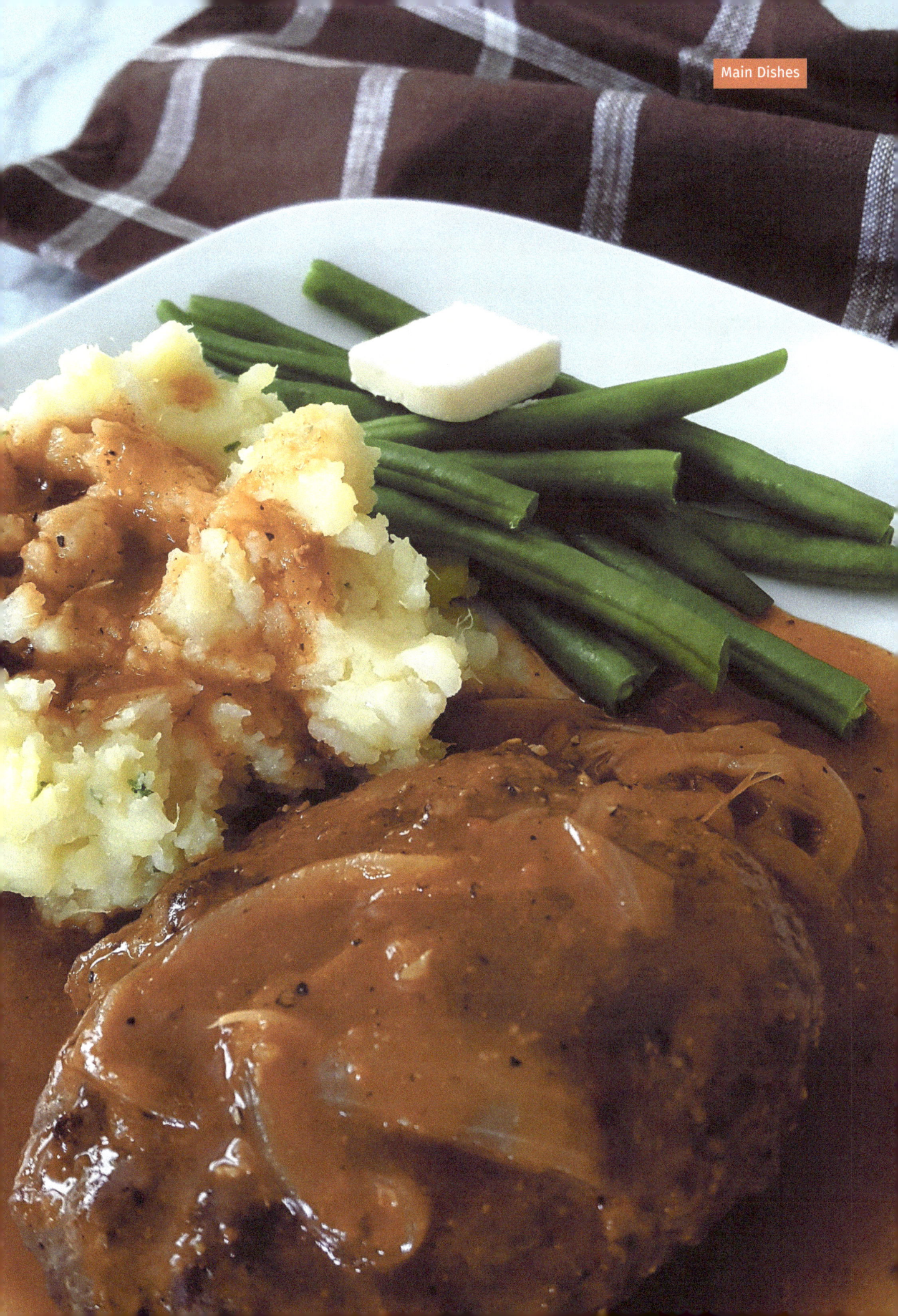

COMFORT COOKING
for Bariatric Post-Ops and Everyone Else!

MOM'S HUNGARIAN BEEF STEW

My mom is Hungarian, and we were basically raised on meat and potatoes. This loving stew is her signature recipe that results in tender beef nuggets blanketed in a velvety soft gravy.

INGREDIENTS

- 1 T. olive oil
- 1½ lb. Chuck roast (cut into 1½ inch cubes)
- 2 medium onions, chopped
- 3 T. sweet paprika
- 2 packets beef bouillon (I use Knorr OXO)
- ¼ t. black pepper
- 2 t. salt
- ½ t. garlic powder
- ¼ t. or more cayenne pepper if you like a kick
- 8 oz. white flesh sweet potato, cubed
- ½ c. water

INSTRUCTIONS

1. In a large soup pot, add oil and onions and cook over very low heat, stirring occasionally, making sure NOT to caramelize. This should take about 15 to 20 minutes, and onions should be soft and glossy.

2. Remove from heat. Add two tablespoons paprika to onions and mix well to dissolve. Add the meat and coat well. Add beef packets salt, pepper, garlic powder, remaining paprika, cayenne pepper, and water. Mix well and return pot to heat.

3. Heat to a low simmer, cover with lid cracked open slightly and continue to cook until meat is fork-tender, about one and a half to two hours. If boil is too rapid, then lower the heat. Visit often and give it a stir.

4. When the meat is super-tender (use the back of a spoon and mush down on a piece of meat), turn off heat and uncover to thicken. Taste and adjust salt and pepper.

5. In a separate pot, boil salted water and add potatoes. Boil for about 11 to 12 minutes, till tender but not mushy. Remove from heat and steam out in the sink for 10 minutes in a colander. When the potatoes no longer appear wet, carefully add them to the stew making sure to distribute all around without mushing them! I use a fork for this!

6. Heat gently to serve.

Main Dishes

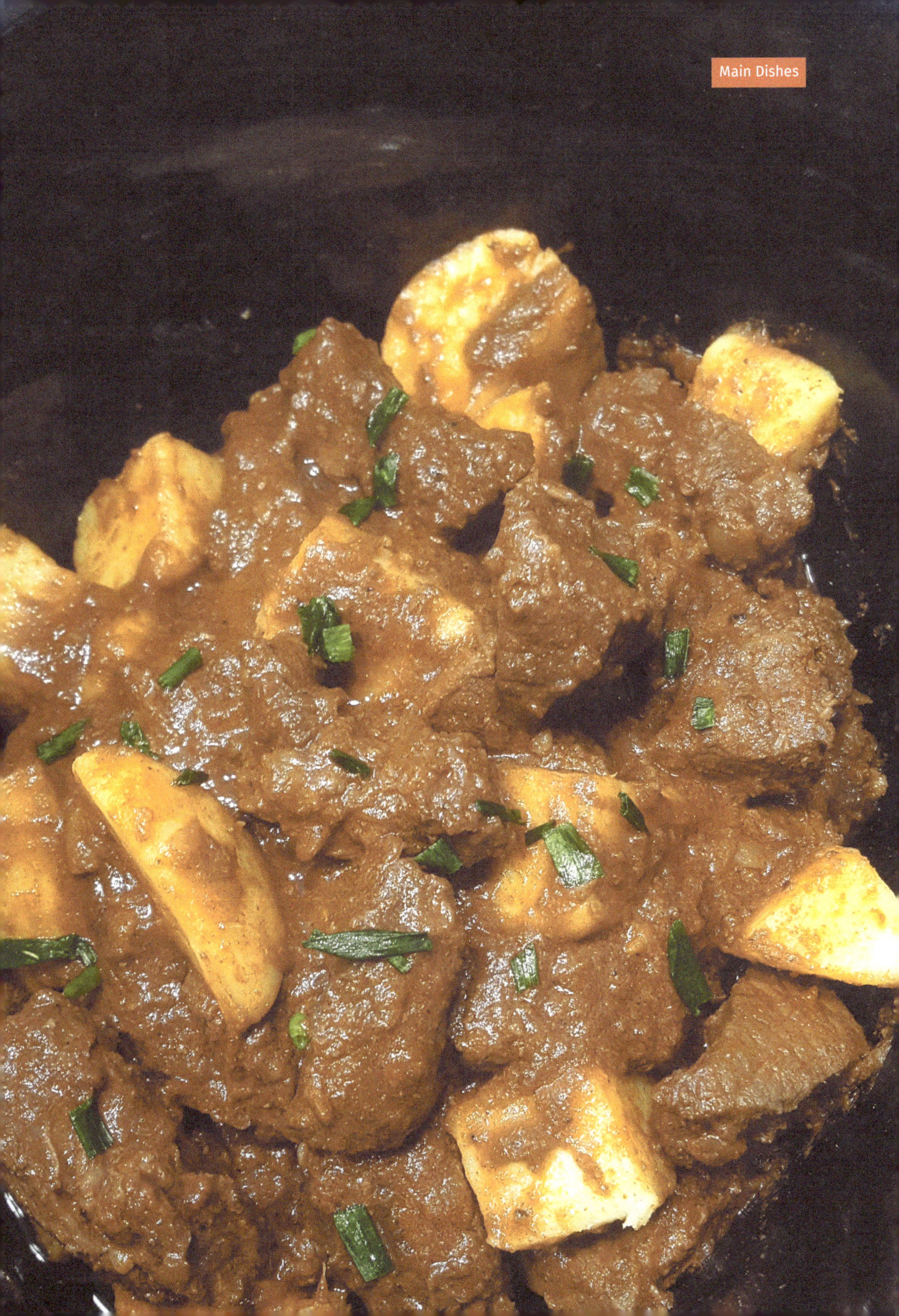

LASAGNA SKILLET

Mom would never buy that box with the mitten on the front. Finally, I figured out how to relive that childhood memory with a happy ending in this healthier remake!

INGREDIENTS

- ½ lb. lean ground beef
- ½ lb. lean Italian sausage
- 1 packet beef bouillon (I use Knorr OXO)
- 1 T. olive oil
- 1 small onion, chopped
- 2 garlic cloves, minced
- ½ t. garlic powder
- 1 t. onion powder
- 1 t. salt
- ¼ t. black pepper
- 1 T. dried Italian seasoning
- 1 T. dried parsley
- 1 t. Truvia Baking Blend
- 1 T. parmesan cheese
- 1 c. reduced-fat combination cheddar/mozzarella cheese, shredded
- 2 c. low-sugar tomato sauce
- ¼ c. milk
- 1 T. butter
- ½ c. low-sodium chicken broth mixed with ½ t. cornstarch
- ½ c. reduced-fat ricotta cheese mixed with 1 T. parmesan cheese
- 2 Low-Carb Crêpes, cut into noodle forms (recipe found in Sides)

INSTRUCTIONS

1. In a large skillet, over medium heat, sauté onions and garlic in olive oil for 10 minutes, until softened. Add meat, seasonings, Truvia, and one tablespoon parmesan and cook until browned and well combined.
2. Add tomato sauce, milk, butter, and broth. Mix well.
3. Cover and simmer on low for 12 to 15 minutes. Remove from heat and stir in cheese till it melts.
4. Gently fold in "noodles" and distribute all around. Serve topped with a dollop of ricotta!

NOTE: You can make classic-style lasagna using this recipe with a few extra crêpes and layering in an 8 × 8 glass baking dish (see my Beef Enchilada recipe and follow the layering technique, substituting with lasagna meat).

Main Dishes

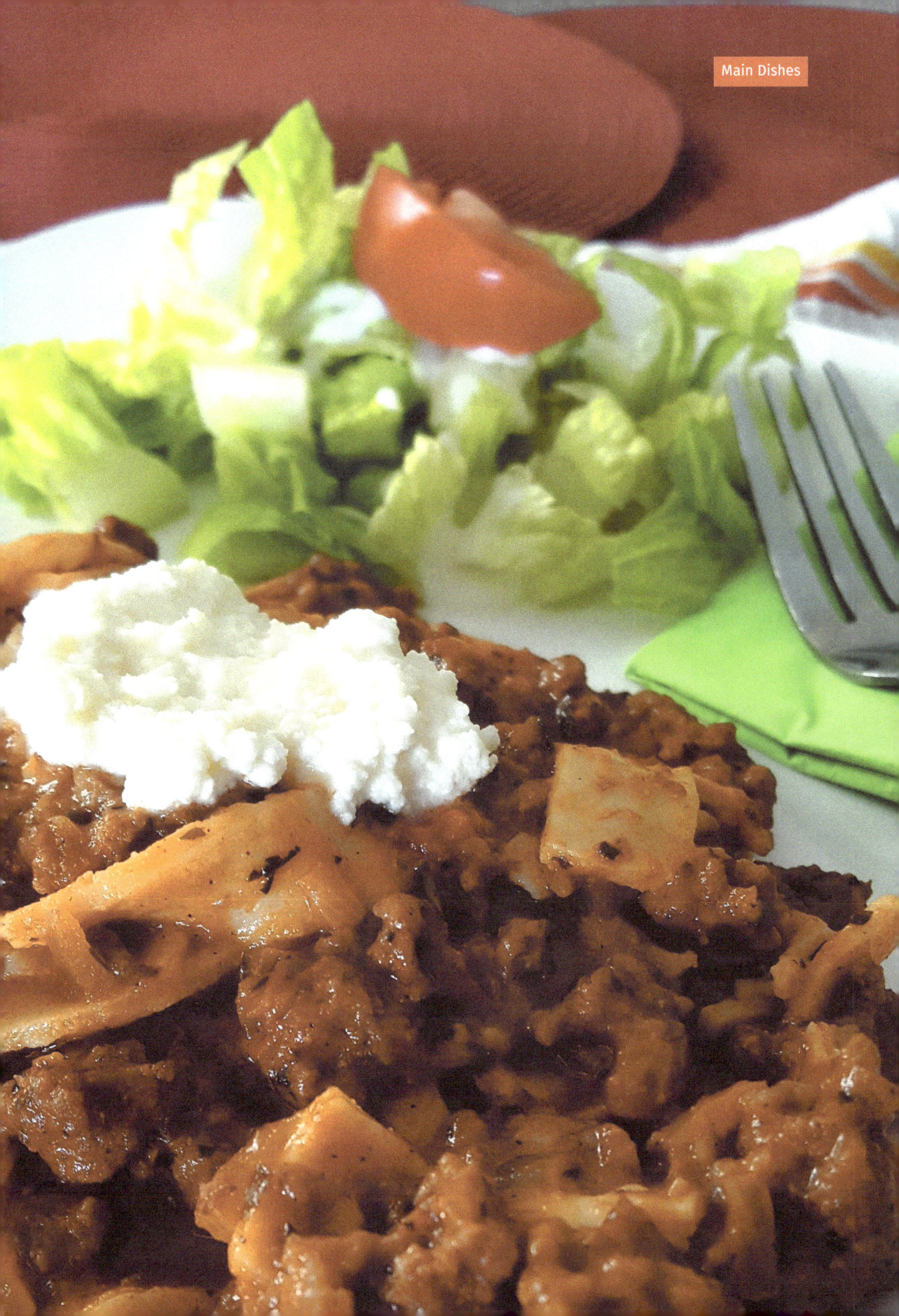

CHILI MAC SKILLET

Another variation of the boxed oven mitt. Tasty and on the table in no time!

INGREDIENTS

- 1 lb. lean ground beef
- 1 T. olive oil
- 1 small onion, chopped
- 1 t. garlic powder
- 1 t. salt
- 1 t. onion powder
- ½ t. oregano
- ¼ t. black pepper
- 2 packets beef bouillon (I use Knorr OXO)
- 1½ T. chili powder
- ¼ t. cayenne pepper
- ¼ t. paprika
- 1 shake Tabasco sauce
- 1 shake Worcestershire sauce
- 1 T. lemon juice
- 1 T. low-sugar tomato sauce
- 1 ½ c. low-sodium beef broth mixed with 2 t. cornstarch
- ½ c. reduced-fat cheddar cheese, shredded
- 1 t. nacho cheese flavoured popcorn seasoning
- 2 Low-Carb Crêpes, cut into noodle forms (recipe found in Sides)

INSTRUCTIONS

1. In a large skillet, over medium heat, sauté onion in olive oil until softened, about 10 minutes. Add ground beef and all spices. Brown until cooked through.
2. Add Tabasco, Worcestershire, lemon juice, tomato sauce, and broth and cook an additional 10 minutes over medium–low heat.
3. Remove from heat and add the cheese, stirring until melted and well combined. Add the popcorn seasoning. Taste and adjust salt and pepper.
4. Gently add the noodles and distribute evenly. Enjoy!

Main Dishes

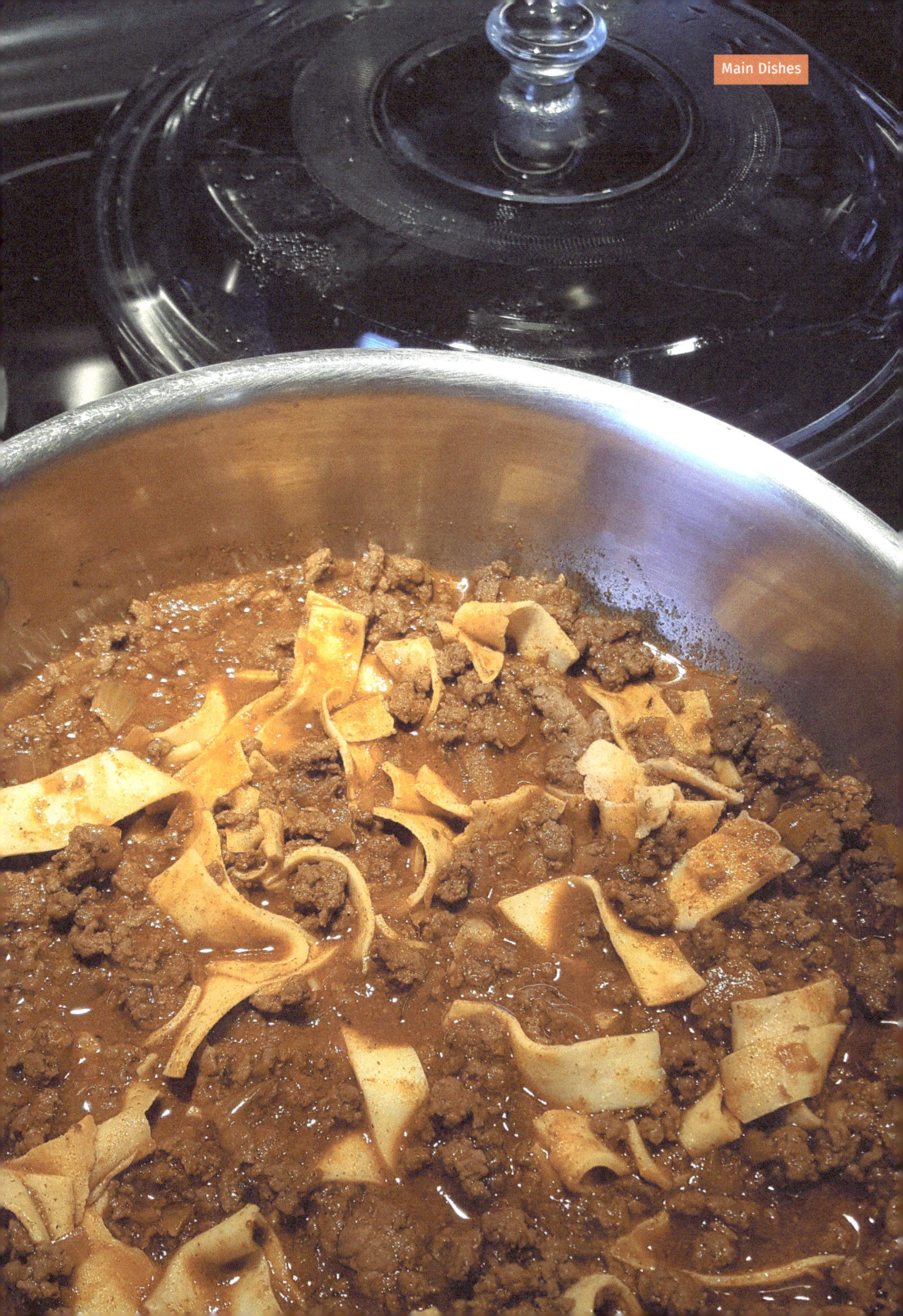

BEEF STROGANOFF CRÊPES

My Low-Carb Crêpes are so very versatile. There is a slight difference between the crêpes used for dessert and the crêpes used for savory dishes like this one. Whatever the case may be, keep a bunch of each ready in the freezer to enjoy the many recipes in this book.

INGREDIENTS

Makes about six or seven crêpes

- 1 lb. lean ground beef
- 1 t. olive oil
- 1 t. butter
- ¼ c. onions, chopped
- 6 oz. white mushrooms, sliced
- ½ t. garlic powder
- ½ t. onion powder
- ½ t. salt
- ¼ t. black pepper
- ¼ c. low-sodium beef broth
- 1 packet beef bouillon (I use Knorr OXO)
- 1 packet brown gravy, mixed with 1 c. water (I use Knorr classic brown)
- ¼ c. 0% plain Greek yogurt
- 6 or 7 Low-Carb Crêpes (recipe found in Sides)

INSTRUCTIONS

1. In a large skillet, heat olive oil and butter over medium–low heat. When foamy, add onions and cook until transparent, about 10 minutes. Add mushrooms and cook 10 minutes longer.
2. Add spices, beef broth, bouillon, and gravy. Bring to a boil.
3. Reduce heat to medium, and add the ground beef to the gravy, breaking it up with a wooden spoon as it cooks through. About 10 to 12 minutes.
4. Cook for an additional five minutes while it thickens as moisture is released. Remove from heat and mix in the yogurt.
5. Fill each crêpe in the middle with about one-quarter cup of filling and fold each end toward the centre, overlapping them. Garnish each crêpe with a dollop of warmed yogurt, thinned out with beef broth.

Main Dishes

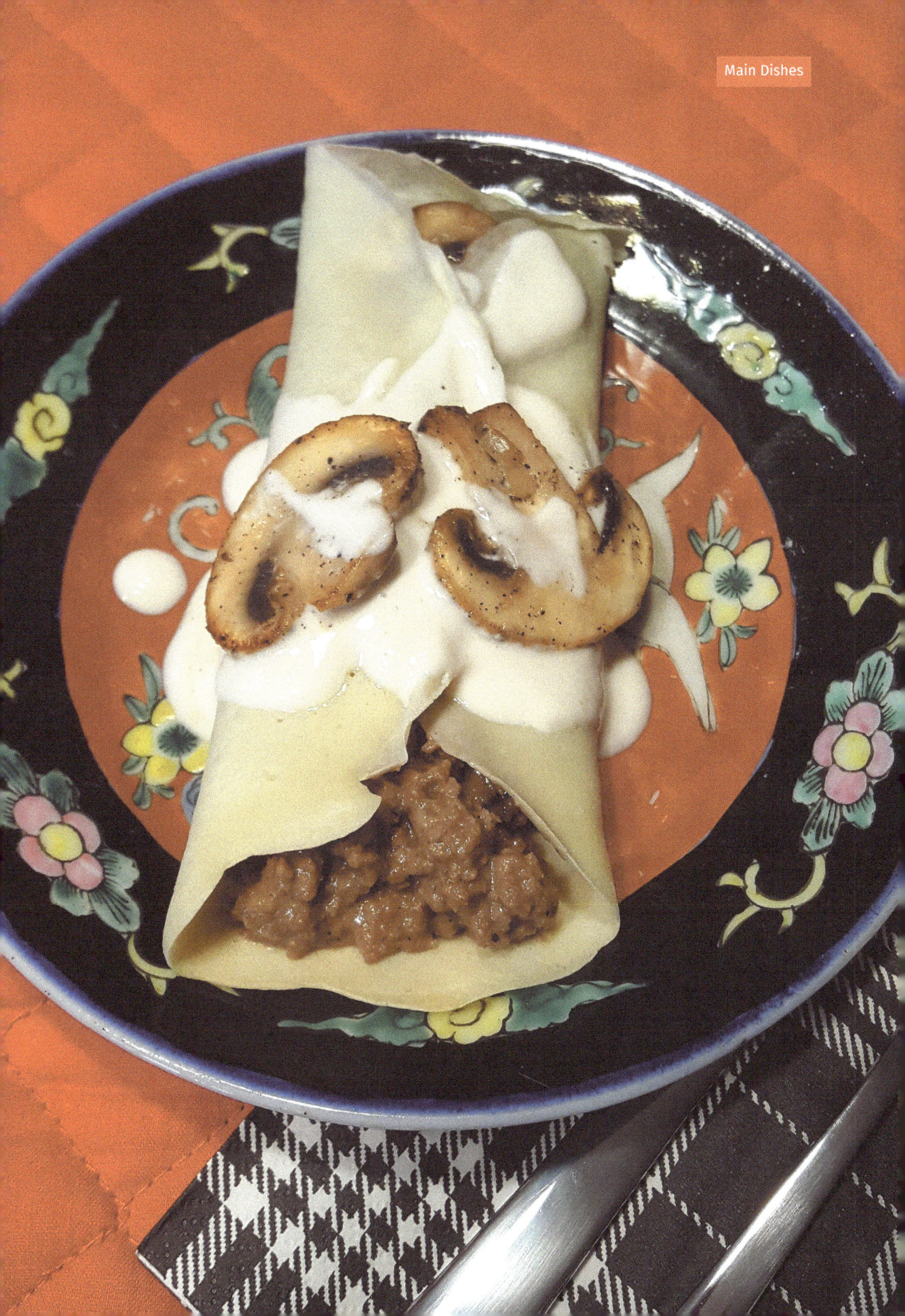

COMFORT COOKING
for Bariatric Post-Ops and Everyone Else!

SLOW COOKER PULLED POT ROAST

Decades ago, when I got my first slow cooker, I hardly used it. After bariatric surgery, it became my new best friend. To make any meat extra-tender and flavourful, it's got to be low and slow. This recipe was inspired by Louisa, my best friend since grade school, who is well known for her wonderful pot roasts.

INGREDIENTS

2–3 lb. boneless Chuck (preferably) roast, string removed

¼ t. ground black pepper

1½ t. garlic powder

1 T. melted butter

½ c. low-sodium beef stock

Montreal steak spice (I use Club House La Grille)

INSTRUCTIONS

1. Spray the cooking pot with vegetable spray. Set out your spices and other ingredients and have them measured and ready to go. Just open the lid of the steak spice, as you will be shaking it in from the container.

2. Place the roast into the slow cooker, fat side down, and rub the melted butter all over the meat in every direction including underneath. (I put disposable kitchen latex gloves on for this.)

3. Shake on the pepper and garlic powder and then the steak spice, making sure you shake it all over the roast. Be sure to go easy on the steak spice as it is fairly salty. Remember, you can always add more later on.

4. Add beef stock by pouring it from the inner edge of the pot. Cover and set the temperature to "high" for four hours. Baste every hour if possible. After four hours, turn temperature to "low" and cook for another three hours, basting every hour if possible. Check meat after the three hours, and, if you feel it needs longer, then cook an additional hour to hour and a half. This is not an exact science as some cuts of meat need longer.

5. Remove meat onto a large plate. Meat should be soft enough to flake when pulled with a fork.

6. Using two forks, pull the meat in opposite directions to shred. Continue shredding until you are finished. Return the meat and any juices to the slow cooker, and, if you think it should be softer, go for another hour on low. Taste and add more steak spice, if necessary.

7. Smother meat with your choice of gravy or sauce (recipes found in Gravy and Sauces). I personally like my pulled roast with my Mushroom Gravy, but my No-Sugar BBQ Sauce comes in a close second.

Main Dishes

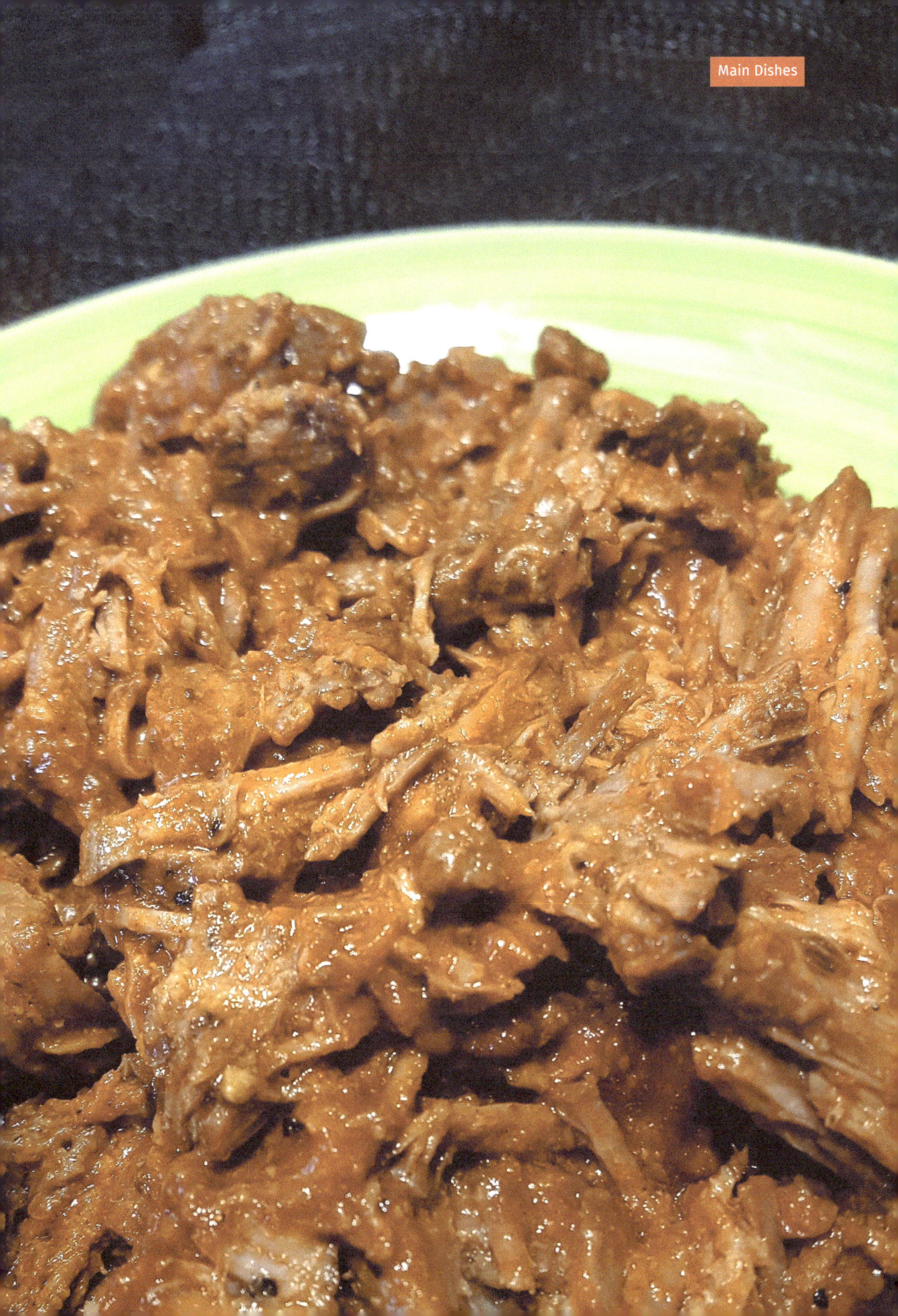

GENERAL TSO'S CHICKEN MAKEOVER

For many families, a weekly visit to a Chinese restaurant was tradition. More than ever, we are aware of the amount of sugar and fat that goes into making most of our favourite dishes. Here is an all-time favourite dish made over. Tastes even better than the restaurant kind! Serve it over Fried "Rice"!

INGREDIENTS

- 1 t. sesame oil
- 1 large egg white
- ¼ c. plus 1 T. soy sauce
- 3 T. cornstarch
- 1 lb. boneless skinless chicken thighs, cut into bite-sized pieces
- 1 c. low-sodium chicken broth
- 1 t. Chinese chili garlic sauce
- 3 T. granular sweetener (or half the amount of Truvia Baking Blend)
- 1½ T. vegetable oil
- 1 T. white vinegar
- ¼ t. hot chili flakes
- 2 T. fresh ginger, chopped
- 2 garlic cloves, minced
- 4 green onions, sliced thinly

INSTRUCTIONS

1. In a medium-sized bowl, whisk together sesame oil, egg white, one tablespoon soy sauce, and two tablespoons cornstarch. Add chicken pieces and toss to coat. Set aside for 20 minutes at room temperature.

2. In a separate bowl, mix together chicken broth, chili garlic sauce, sweetener, remaining one-quarter cup soy sauce, vinegar, remaining one tablespoon cornstarch, and chili flakes.

3. In a medium-sized skillet over medium–high heat, sauté the ginger and garlic in one-half tablespoon vegetable oil for one to two minutes until softened. Add broth to pan and cook till thickened and glossy, between three to five minutes. Set aside and keep warm.

4. In a large-sized non-stick skillet, heat one tablespoon oil over medium–high heat and add the chicken pieces, one by one, making sure not to crowd. Cook till brown and crisp on both sides (three to four minutes per side). Make sure chicken is cooked through.

5. Add the chicken pieces to the warm sauce and toss to coat. Garnish with green onions and it's ready to serve!

Main Dishes

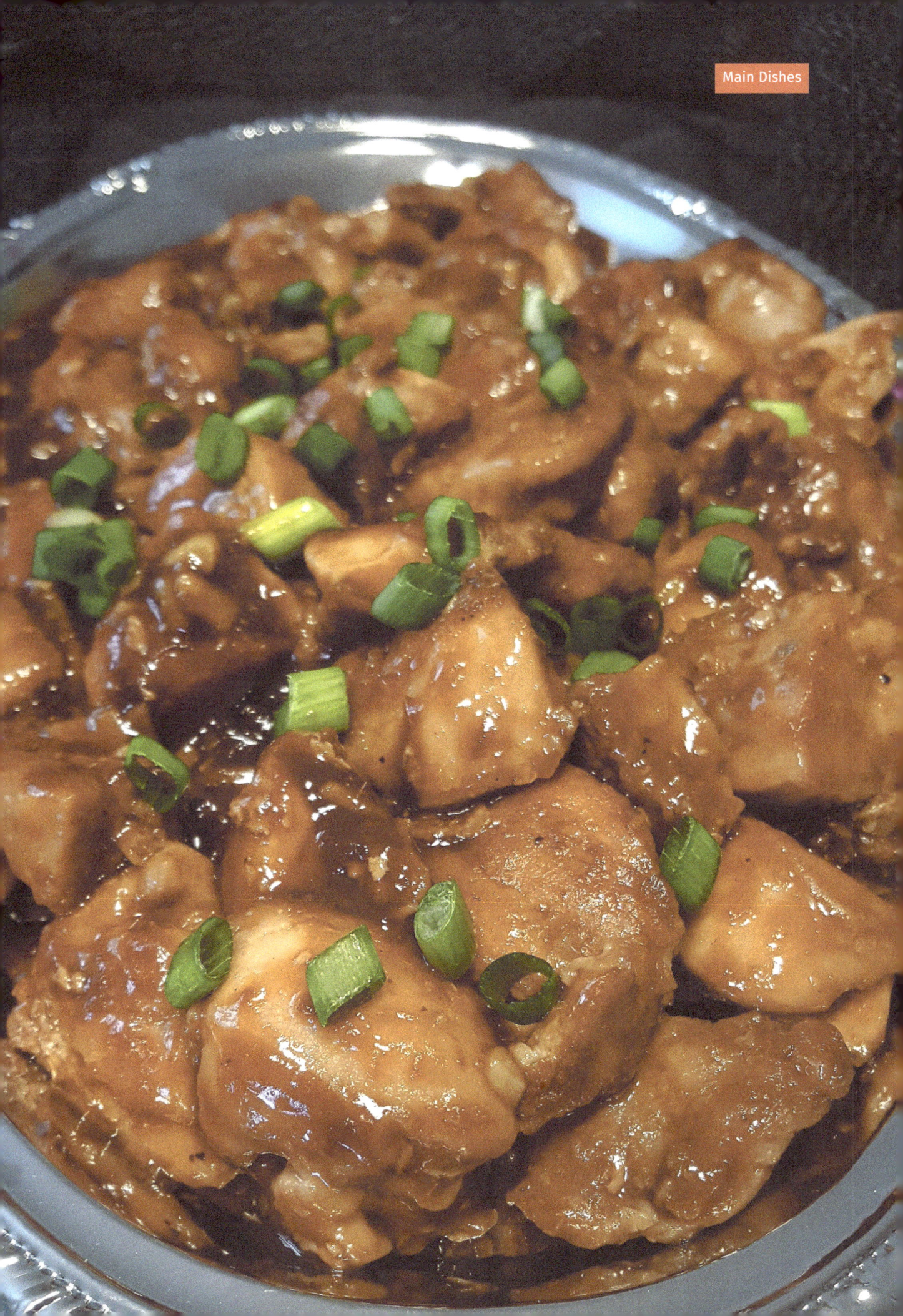

COMFORT COOKING
for Bariatric Post-Ops and Everyone Else!

CHICKEN POT PIE

I love this recipe. There is really nothing more to say. The picture says it all. Enjoy.

INGREDIENTS

½ c. low-fat milk

¾ c. low-sodium chicken broth

1 envelope turkey or chicken gravy mix (I use Knorr classic turkey)

½ t. dried thyme

½ t. poultry seasoning

¼ t. ground black pepper

2½ c. rotisserie chicken, cubed

2 c. frozen mixed vegetables, boiled to soften

2 green onions, thinly sliced

2 T. parmesan cheese

INSTRUCTIONS

1. In a large saucepan, combine milk, broth, gravy mix, thyme, poultry seasoning, and pepper. Bring to a boil, stirring constantly till thickened and smooth.

2. Reduce heat to low and stir in chicken, vegetables, and onions. Simmer for five to eight minutes, stirring occasionally, till hot and bubbly. Remove from heat and stir in parmesan cheese.

3. Serve in a deep bowl with or without the "Topper."

THE TOPPER

1 c. almond flour

½ t. garlic powder

½ t. dried thyme

¼ t. salt

A dash of ground black pepper

½ T. plus ½ t. water

1½ T. olive oil.

Pre-heat oven to 400°F.

1. In a small bowl, combine almond flour, garlic powder, dried thyme, salt, ground black pepper, water, and olive oil. The dough will be very crumbly.

2. With clean hands, press the dough out as evenly as possible into a square in an ungreased 9 × 9 baking pan. It will not fill the entire pan. With a knife, score the dough into nine squares. Bake till crust is golden and firm to the touch, about 10 to 12 minutes. Allow to cool and carefully separate the squares. Top off your Chicken Pot Pie! You will have leftover squares to freeze. However, I usually double the recipe so I have plenty frozen. Use a larger pan if you decide to double the recipe.

Main Dishes

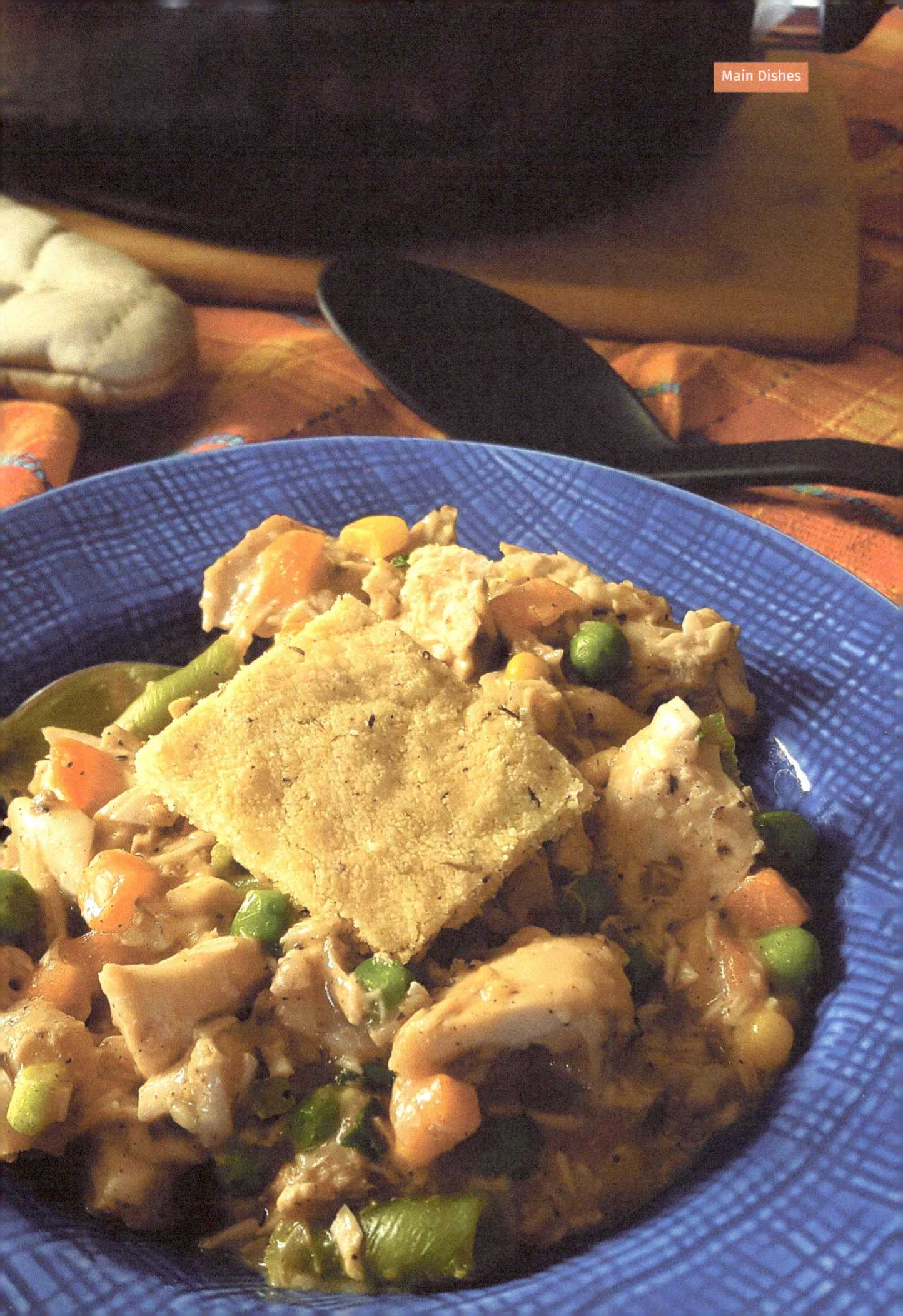

COMFORT CHICKEN BOWL

One of my favourite things that I used to order at that fast-food place. This one is every bit as tasty without all the bad carbs and fat. I no longer pine for the Colonel's version.

INGREDIENTS

Serves one

- 1 c. rotisserie chicken, cubed
- 1 c. Faux Mashed "Potatoes" (recipe found in Sides)
- Chicken Gravy (recipe found in Gravy and Sauces)
- 2 oz. reduced-fat cheddar cheese, shredded
- Extra seasonings: dried thyme, black pepper, poultry seasoning

TO ASSEMBLE

1. Get your favourite microwave-safe soup bowl. We are just going to layer the ingredients.
2. Add chicken and a pinch of fresh black pepper, a pinch of thyme, and a pinch of poultry seasoning over it.
3. Ladle some gravy (about one-quarter cup) over the chicken and then place the Faux Mashed "Potatoes" over the chicken. Put the cheese over the "potatoes" and another ladle of gravy over the cheese.
4. Microwave on high for two minutes, until hot and bubbly. Serve immediately!

Main Dishes

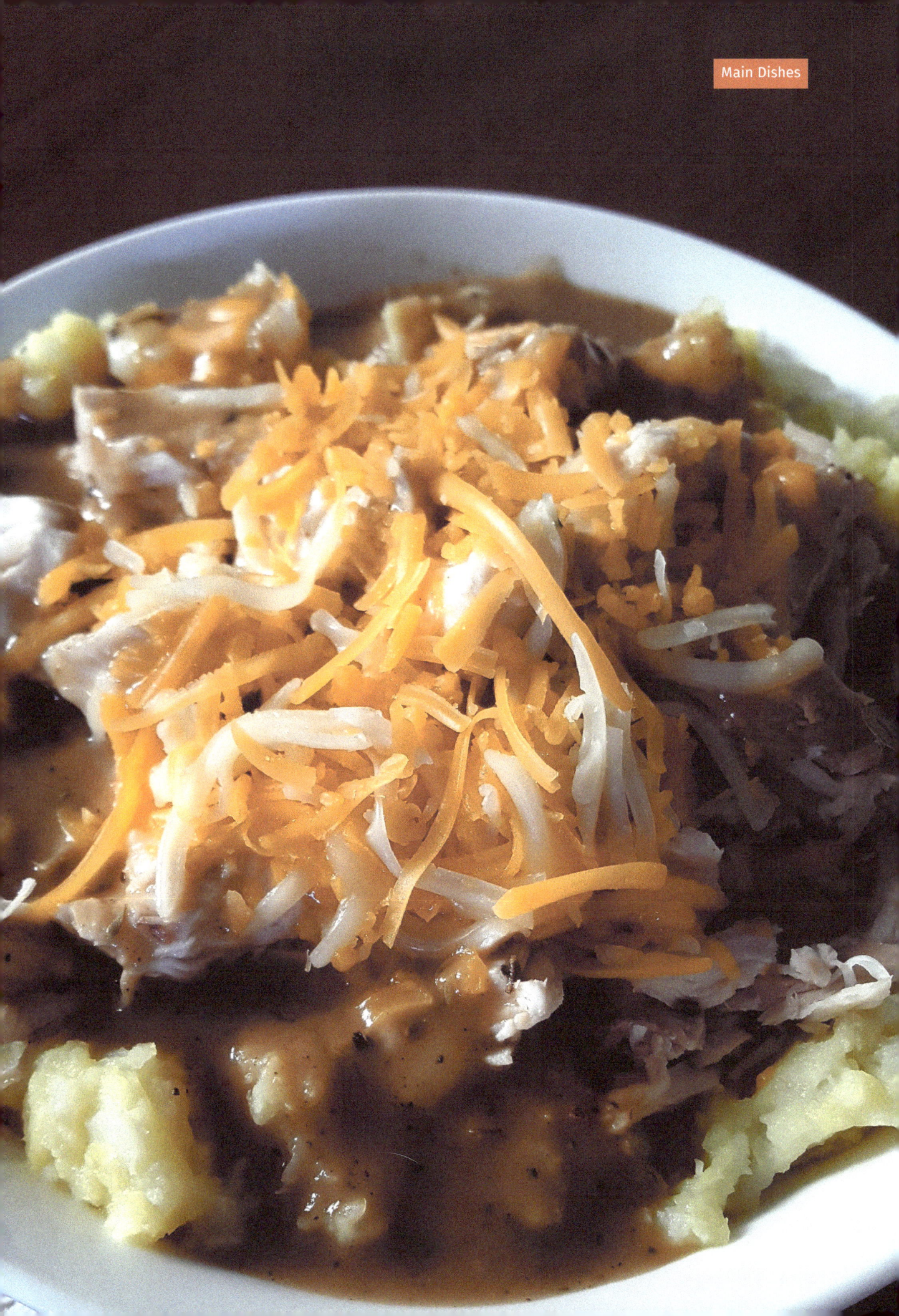

CRISPY CHICKEN FINGERS

Make either strips or nuggets. This is a winner recipe that you will enjoy every time you make it. There is a bit of prep work involved, but it is highly worth it! Do not worry about the small amount of panko or flour. For the portion you will be eating, it will not bring on the carb cravings.

INGREDIENTS

- ⅓ c. panko bread crumbs
- ¼ c. parmesan cheese
- ¼ t. garlic powder
- ¼ t. ground black pepper
- ½ t. salt
- 1½ T. flour
- 2 eggs, beaten
- 2 large boneless skinless chicken breasts, cut into strips or nuggets
- 3 T. olive oil

INSTRUCTIONS

1. Put the first five ingredients into a large plastic Ziploc bag. Seal the bag, give it a shake and set aside.
2. Cut the chicken into strips or nuggets. Sprinkle a pinch of salt, pepper, and garlic powder over them.
3. Measure out the flour onto a flat dish and place the beaten egg next to it in a bowl.
4. Dredge the pieces of chicken by hand, <u>very</u> lightly into the flour, one by one, shaking the excess off. Place onto a plate.
5. Dip the chicken pieces into the egg, then place the meat into the bag of coating. Shake well to distribute. Remove the chicken from the bag and place onto a plate. Cover with plastic wrap and place in the fridge for one hour. Discard the Ziploc bag to the trash.
6. Heat up a non-stick skillet with oil over medium–high heat, and when the oil is good and hot, you are ready to pan fry the chicken pieces. Each side will need about three to four minutes, depending on the thickness. Use a mesh guard to avoid hot oil splatters. Flip with tongs after four minutes and cook the second side. Make sure the chicken is cooked through. Drain on paper towel and serve immediately with Ranch Dipping Sauce, mustard, or no-sugar-added ketchup. Enjoy!

RANCH DIPPING SAUCE

- 1 c. 0% plain Greek yogurt
- 2 t. reduced-fat mayonnaise
- ½ envelope ranch dressing powder (I use Hidden Valley)

Main Dishes

INSTRUCTIONS

1. Combine yogurt, mayonnaise, and ranch dressing powder.
2. Thin with a little milk, if desired.

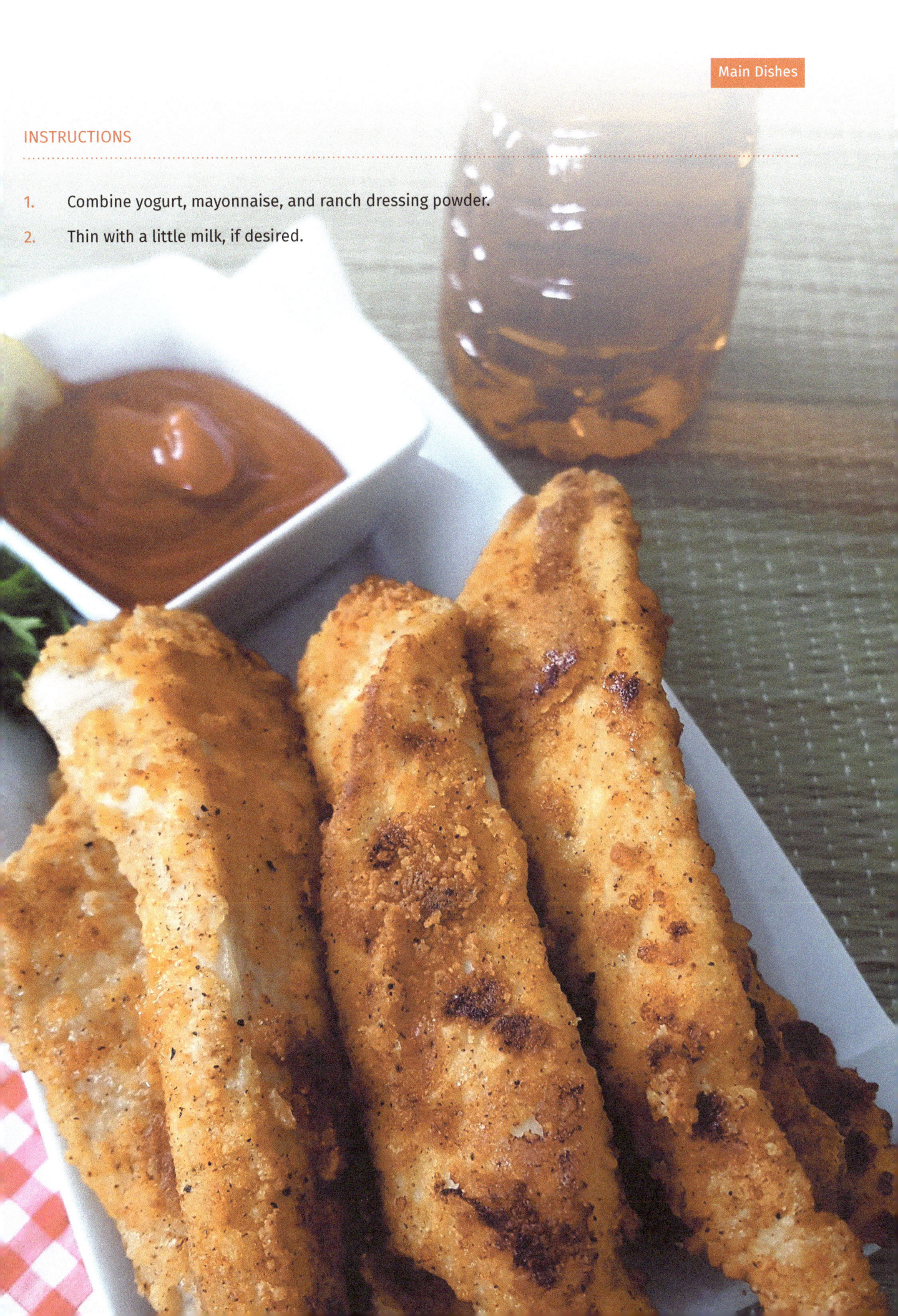

BBQ RIBS

Fall-off-the-bone tender, with finger-licking good No-Sugar BBQ Sauce. This is a match made in heaven!

INGREDIENTS

1 or 2 racks pork back ribs, each cut into 3–4 rib pieces

Seasoned salt (I use Hy's seasoning salt)

Ground black pepper and garlic powder

1–2 c. or more No-Sugar BBQ Sauce (recipe found in Gravy and Sauces)

¼ c. water

Liquid smoke

Sugar-free maple syrup (optional)

BBQ sauce for basting before serving

INSTRUCTIONS

Pre-heat oven to 350°F.

1. Spray an oven roaster large enough to accommodate the ribs with vegetable spray. Arrange the ribs in the roaster and sprinkle the raw ribs with seasoning salt, garlic powder, and black pepper. Make sure that the undersides are also seasoned.

2. Mix the water into the BBQ sauce and pour over the ribs. Cover and bake for two and a half to three hours.

3. Re-visit the ribs every hour to baste. If the ribs appear in need of more liquid, add one-quarter cup of water to the roaster and baste to distribute.

4. When ribs are fall-off-the-bone tender, remove from the oven, give a few shakes of liquid smoke and a drizzle of maple syrup over the meat. Taste the sauce, and if you feel it needs more salt, give it a light shake of seasoned salt. Baste one more time just before serving with more sauce.

5. Enjoy with Coleslaw or Caesar Salad and Twice-Baked Loaded "Potatoes"—all found in this book!

Main Dishes

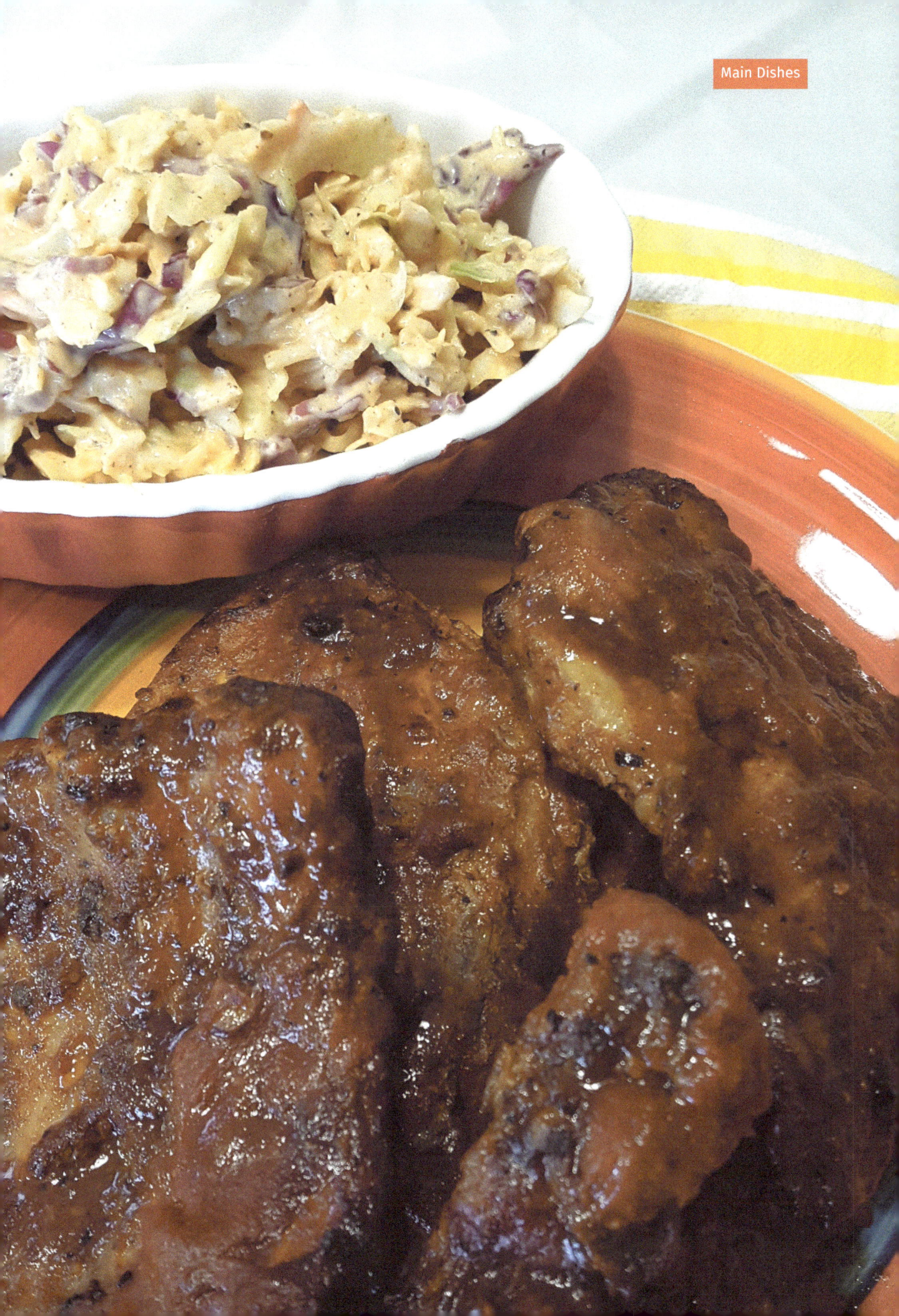

COMFORT COOKING
for Bariatric Post-Ops and Everyone Else!

SURPRISE PIZZA CRUST

This crust is A-M-A-Z-I-N-G! And nobody but you has to know its magical secret! Smiles everyone!

INGREDIENTS

NOTE: The recipe below is for one 9-inch pie. Make two or three pies for larger families.

- ⅓ c. baking mix (like Bisquick original)
- 1 t. baking powder
- Pinch salt
- ½ t. dried Italian seasoning
- 1 T. parmesan cheese
- ½ t. olive oil
- ¼ c. reduced-fat mozzarella cheese, shredded
- ¼ c. ground chicken, raw
- 1 egg

INSTRUCTIONS

Pre-heat oven to 400°F.

1. Line a 9-inch pie plate with parchment paper sprayed with vegetable spray. Combine ingredients in a medium-sized bowl and mix till well blended.

2. Spoon the mixture onto the centre of the pie plate, then spray a spatula and use it to spread the "dough" thinly to resemble a crust. If you see gaps, fill them in with a bit of mozzarella cheese. Spray the crust with a mist of vegetable spray.

3. Bake for 12 minutes or until lightly browned. Watch so that it does not burn. Remove from oven and let cool for a few minutes. Lift the crust out and remove the parchment paper. Place it back in the pie plate or, if you prefer, a cookie sheet, topside down.

4. Top photo shows result after baking crust (top will become bottom of pie). Bottom photo shows crust flipped and ready to sauce.

5. Proceed to next page for sauce recipe and instruction to assemble and bake your awesome pizza!

Main Dishes

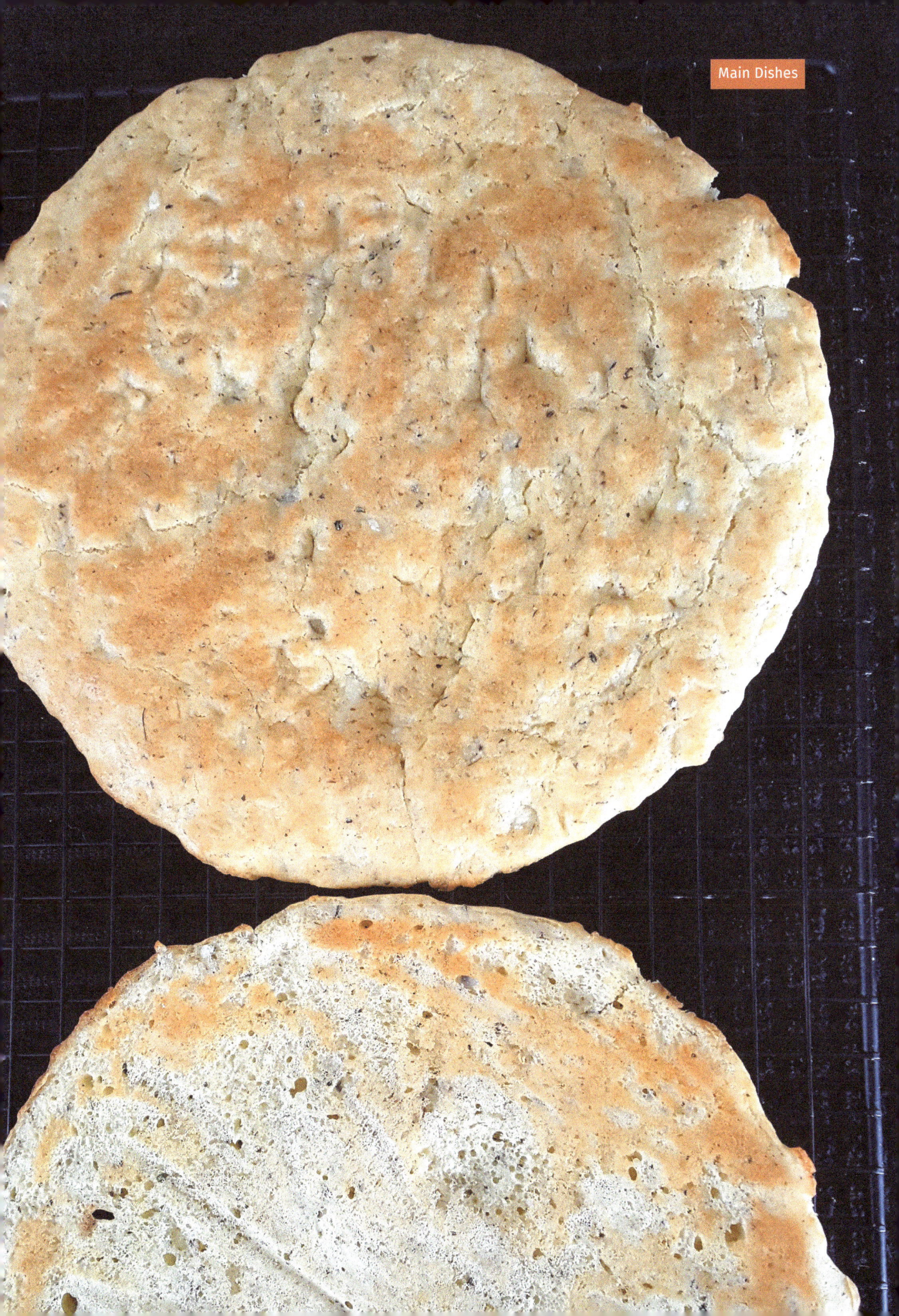

PIZZA!

This pizza is as good, if not better, than any pizza you could order in. Weekly family pizza nights that deliver on taste are back on and EVERYONE is invited!

INGREDIENTS

1 Surprise Pizza Crust (previous recipe)

Pizza Sauce

Pizza Toppings

PIZZA SAUCE

⅓ c. tomato paste

¼ t. garlic powder

1 t. oregano

¼ t. sea salt

½ t. Stevia white granular sweetener

Pinch of black pepper

A few chili flakes

PIZZA TOPPINGS

1 cup reduced fat mozzarella cheese, onions, red peppers, mushrooms, tomatoes, pepperoni, parmesan cheese, dried pepper flakes, etc.

INSTRUCTIONS

Pre-heat oven to 400°F.

1. Place crust topside (brown) down onto pizza plate or cookie sheet.
2. Mix the Pizza Sauce ingredients together in a small bowl, then spoon evenly to cover the crust.
3. Top with Pizza Toppings of your choice.
4. Bake for 10 to 12 minutes or until browned and bubbly!

NOTE: As stated in the previous page's Surprise Pizza Crust recipe, for larger families, plan on preparing at least two crusts!

Main Dishes

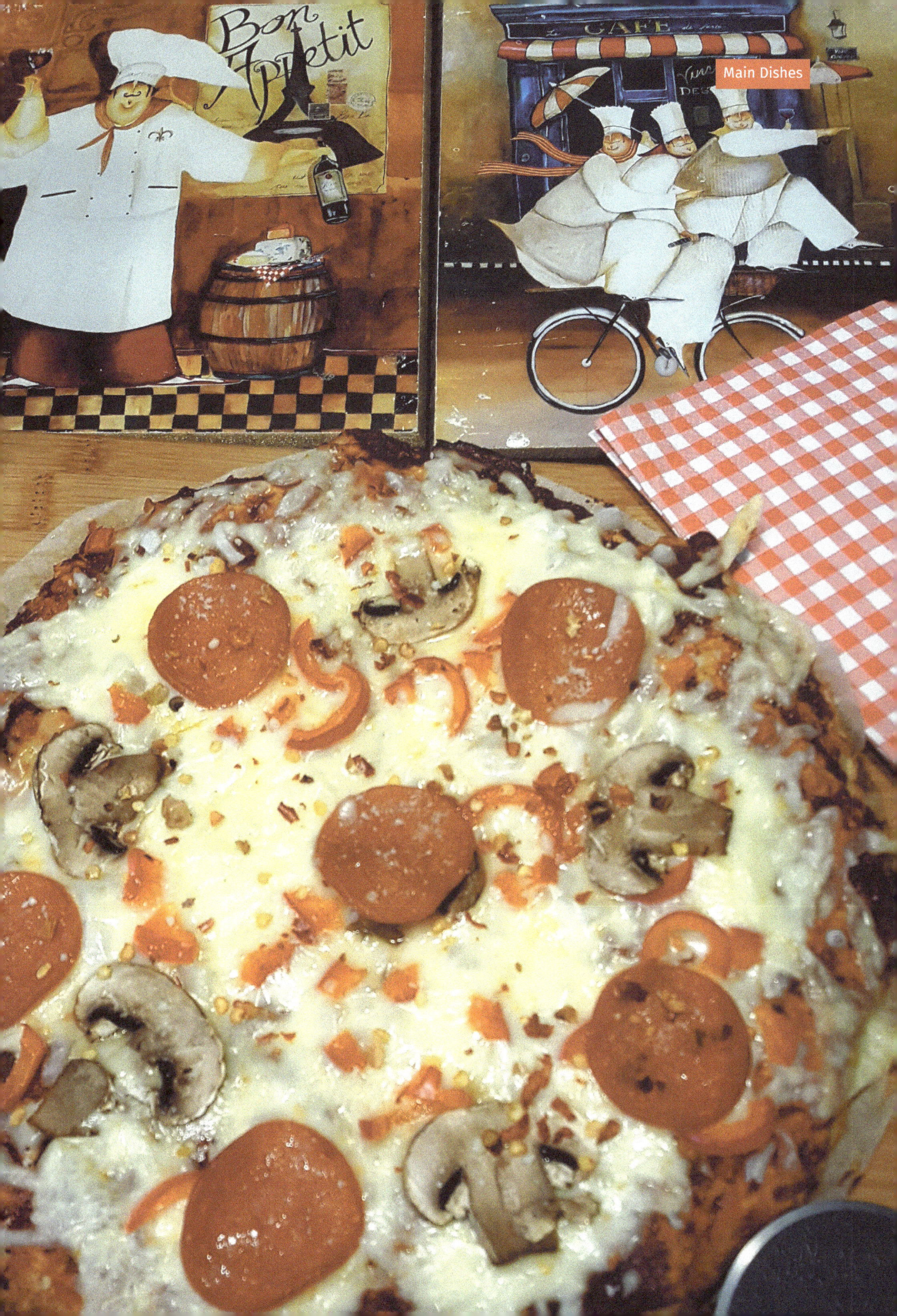

COMFORT COOKING
for Bariatric Post-Ops and Everyone Else!

BROILED CHEESY TUNA CASSEROLE

This is so easy to put together, and it is both creamy and delicious! Dinner can be on the table in less than 25 minutes!

INGREDIENTS

Makes one substantial portion

- 1 T. olive oil
- ¼ c. onion, sliced
- ½ c. fresh broccoli florets (softened in the microwave)
- ¼ c. red pepper, sliced or diced
- 1 can solid white tuna
- Salt and pepper to taste
- ¼ c. Alfredo sauce
- 3 T. reduced-fat cheddar, shredded
- ½ Low-Carb Crêpe, cut into noodle strips (recipe found in Sides)

INSTRUCTIONS

1. In a large skillet, over medium heat, sauté onions, red pepper, and broccoli in olive oil until softened.

2. Turn heat to low and add tuna, carefully breaking it apart into chunks. Combine everything well. Add salt and pepper to taste.

3. Add cut up "noodles" carefully with a fork, distributing them all around. Remove from heat and transfer into an oven-proof dish sprayed with vegetable spray. Pour Alfredo sauce evenly over the mixture and top with shredded cheese. Broil in oven for several minutes till hot, bubbly, and browned.

Main Dishes

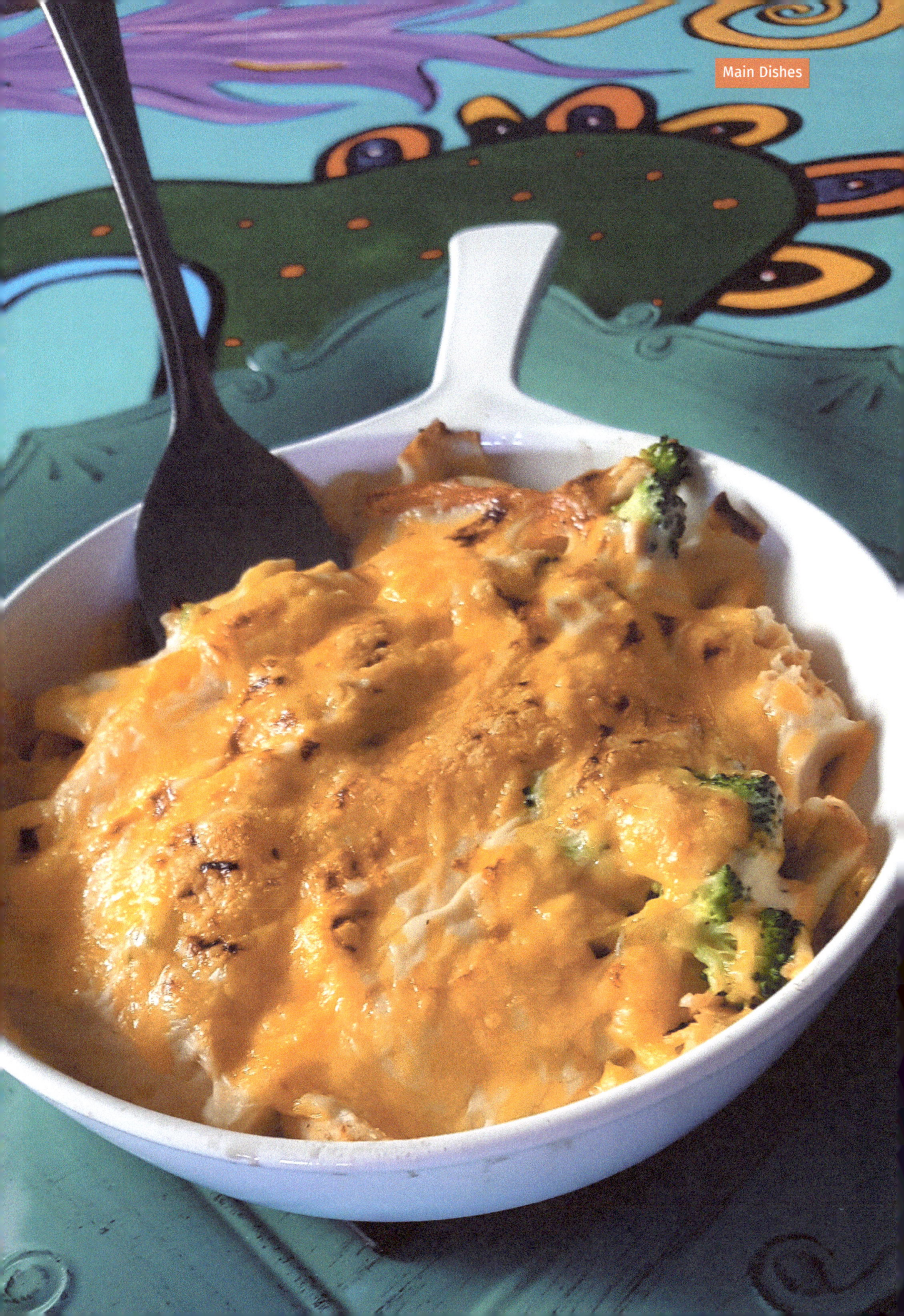

ALFREDO (SHRIMP/CHICKEN)

Who can resist a creamy, garlicky sauce that coats thick zucchini noodles mixed in with strips of "pasta" noodles made out of a Low-Carb Crêpe?

SAUCE INGREDIENTS

- 6 wedges light processed cheese (I use Laughing Cow Light)
- ¼ c. any jarred Alfredo sauce
- 1 t. reduced-fat Caesar salad dressing (I use Renée's)
- ¼ c. low-sodium chicken broth
- ¼ c. parmesan cheese
- 1 t. garlic powder
- Fresh ground pepper to taste

MAIN INGREDIENTS

- 16 medium-sized shrimp, raw and dried with a paper towel
- 2 small zucchinis spiraled into thick noodles (I use a Veggetti)
- 3 garlic cloves, minced
- 1 t. butter
- 1 t. olive oil
- 2 Low-Carb Crêpes (recipe found in Sides), cut into fettuccine-style strips

INSTRUCTIONS

1. Combine Sauce ingredients in a small pot and cook over low heat, stirring frequently until velvety smooth. Remove from heat and set aside.

2. In a large skillet, over medium heat, add butter and olive oil and, when bubbly, sauté garlic for a few minutes. Add shrimp and cook for 30 seconds, then flip them and cook until pink coloured, being careful not to overcook. Remove from heat and shake some salt and pepper on them. Transfer into a bowl and set aside.

3. Return skillet back to medium heat and spray it with a little vegetable spray. Add the zucchini noodles and the "fettuccine" noodles and gently toss for a few minutes, just until warmed. Add two tablespoons of the sauce, just to coat the noodles.

4. Gently heat up the sauce and, when warmed, add the shrimp. Do not boil it or cook, otherwise the shrimp will become rubbery. Plate the noodles and ladle on the sauce!

NOTE: If using chicken, cut chicken breast into strips and follow the same steps as for the shrimp. Remember, chicken takes longer to cook than shrimp, so make sure it is cooked through.

Main Dishes

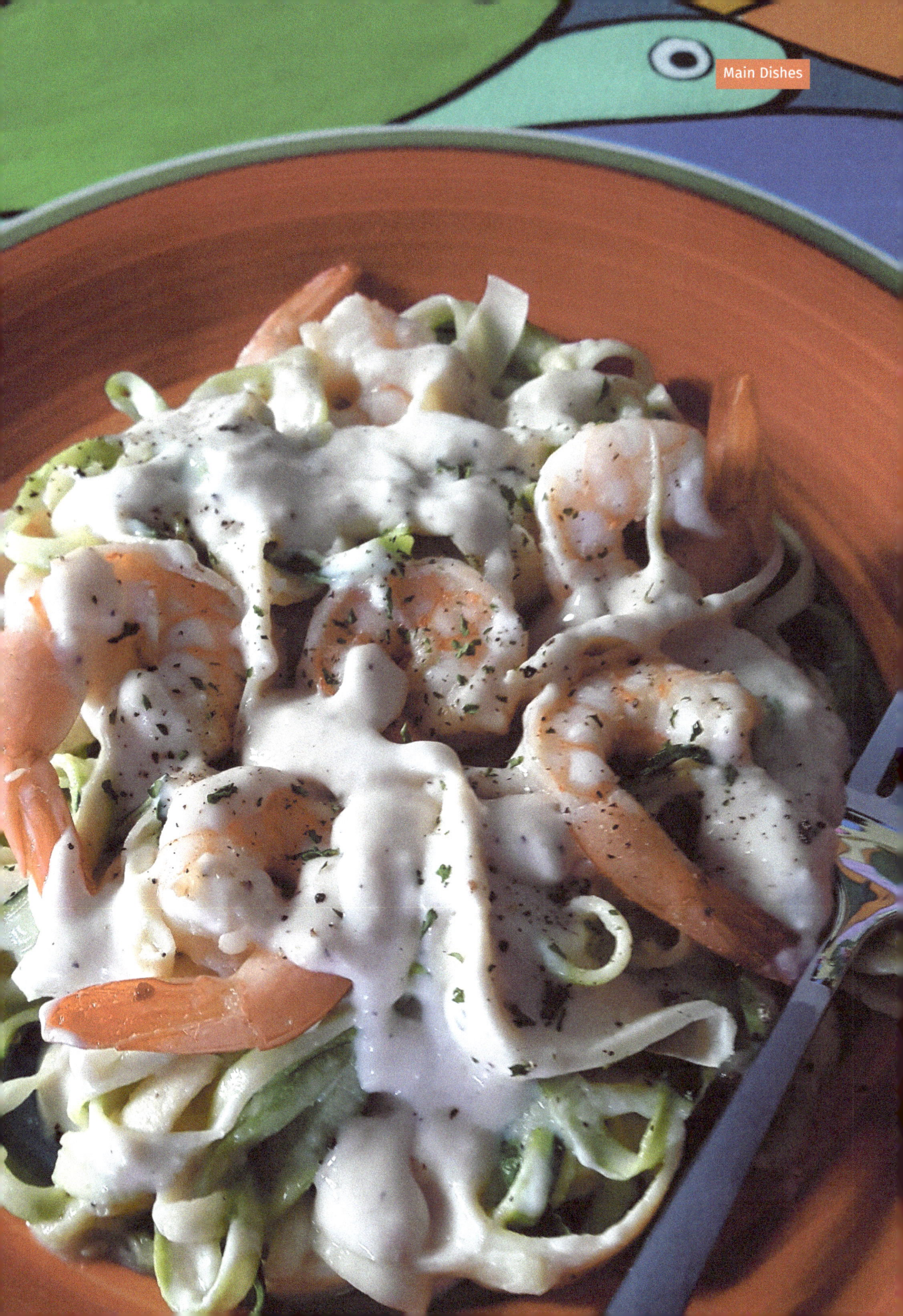

EGG FOO YUNG

A wonderful addition to the other Chinese dishes here. This recipe is quite easy to prepare. Enjoy it on its own, with garlicky shrimp or sweet and sour meatballs, and fried "rice"!

SAUCE INGREDIENTS

- ½ c. low-sodium chicken broth
- ½ c. water
- 1 T. soy sauce
- 2 T. oyster sauce
- 1 T. cornstarch
- 2 garlic cloves, sliced
- ½ t. sesame oil
- ½ t. white vinegar

PANCAKE INGREDIENTS

- 2 T. peanut oil
- 3 green onions, chopped
- ½ c. water chestnuts, diced
- ½ c. mushrooms, sliced
- ¼ c. celery, chopped
- 2 c. bean sprouts
- 1 T. soy sauce
- ½ t. sesame oil
- Ground black pepper to taste
- ½ t. garlic powder
- 1 T. flour
- 6 large eggs

INSTRUCTIONS

1. In a small pot, bring the Sauce ingredients to a boil over high heat, whisking for three minutes, until thickened. Remove from heat and keep sauce warm.

2. Heat one tablespoon peanut oil in a large skillet over medium heat. Sauté onions, water chestnuts, mushrooms, and celery until softened. Add bean sprouts, soy sauce, and sesame oil and toss mixture to combine. Cook a minute longer, just until bean sprouts become limp. Transfer to a bowl and let cool.

3. Wipe the skillet to prepare for the pancakes.

4. In a large bowl, beat the eggs and flour until smooth, then stir in the vegetable mixture.

5. Coat the skillet with the remaining one tablespoon oil and heat up to medium. Ladle one-half cup of the mixture to form a four-inch pancake. Cook for two minutes per side, until golden brown. Continue to make the pancakes until mixture is finished. You should have about 6 pancakes.

6. To serve, spoon warmed sauce over each pancake. Enjoy!

NOTE: To keep the cooked pancakes warm, place them in a 300°F oven while the rest cooks.

Main Dishes

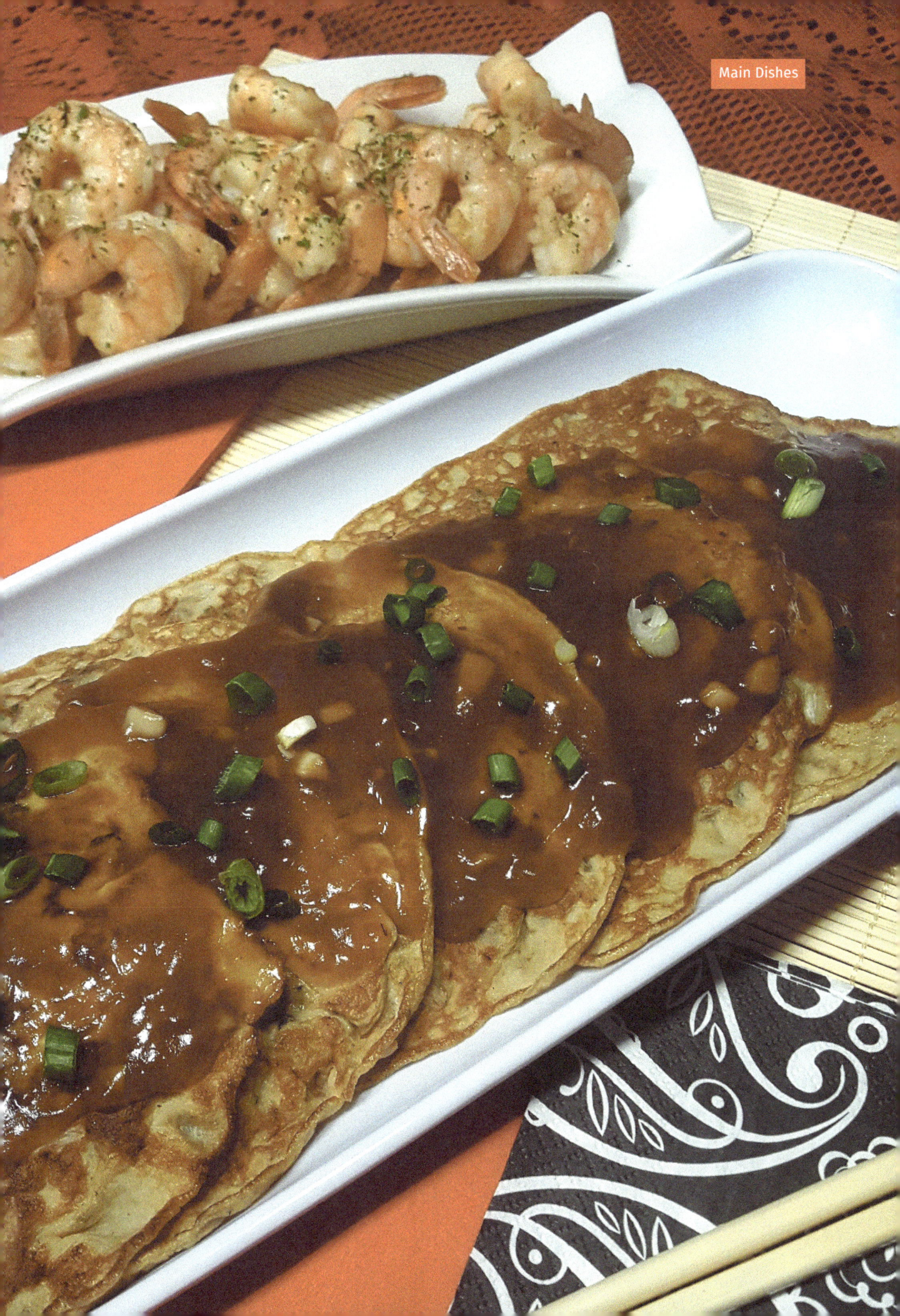

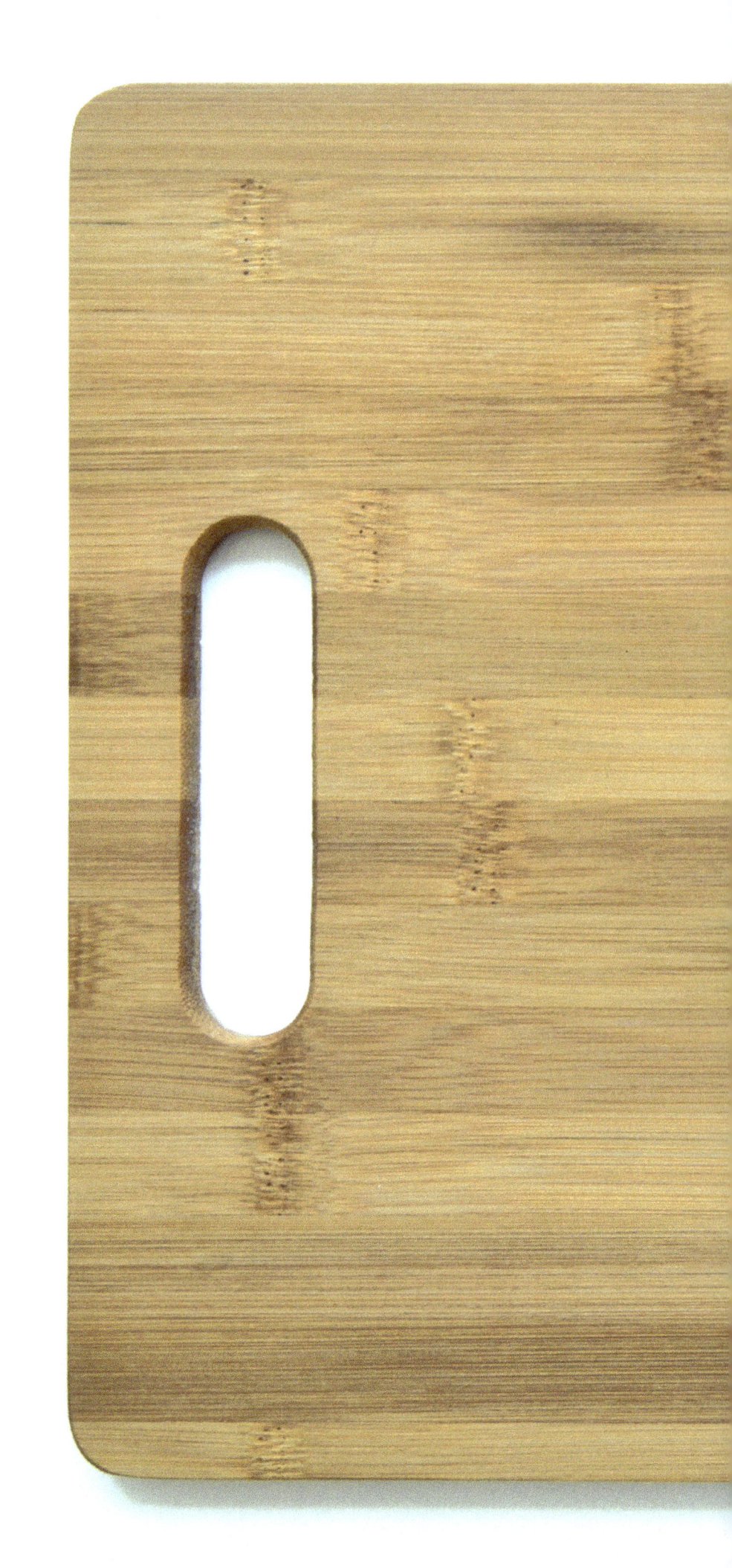

SIDES AND VEGETABLES

"Mac" and Cheese..........................118

Faux Mashed "Potatoes"....................120

Twice-Baked Loaded "Potatoes"............122

Delicious Oven-Baked "Tater" Tots.........124

Fried "Rice"..............................126

Low-Carb "Flatbread" (Because Sometimes You Just Need to Make a Sandwich)........128

Low-Carb Crêpes (Pasta Substitute)........130

Fried Cabbage With Onions and "Pasta" Squares..........................132

Holiday Stuffing..........................134

Cheese Latkes.............................136

Lazy Perogy Casserole.....................138

Roasted Garlicky Brussel Sprouts..........140

Bread and Butter Pickles..................142

Green Bean Casserole Makeover.............144

Spiral Veggie "Noodles"...................146

"MAC" AND CHEESE

We all have fond memories of mac and cheese. Since bariatric surgery, it is a food that is off the list. With a little creative ingenuity, this new bariatric-friendly version is back on the list as a side dish and will satisfy the entire family!

INGREDIENTS

- ½ large cauliflower, cut into about 4 large chunks
- 1¼ c. reduced-fat cheddar cheese, shredded (reserve ¼ c. for topping)
- ½ c. 1% milk plus ¼ c. unsweetened almond milk
- 2 wedges Laughing Cow light cheese
- 1½ t. Dijon mustard
- ¼ t. salt
- ¼ t. black pepper
- ½ t. garlic powder
- 1 t. onion powder
- ½ t. paprika
- Pinch of ground nutmeg
- 1 T. butter (reserve 1 t. for topping)
- 1 t. cheddar cheese popcorn seasoning
- ¼ c. panko bread crumbs
- ¼ c. parmesan cheese
- 1 t. cornstarch, mixed with a little water
- 1 Low-Carb Crêpe (recipe found in Sides)

INSTRUCTIONS

Pre-heat oven to 375°F and prepare an 8 × 8 glass baking dish with vegetable spray.

1. Boil cauliflower in salted water until fork-tender, but not mushy, about 12 minutes. Drain in a colander and allow to steam out for 15 minutes, until most of the moisture is released. Dry off any remaining moisture with a paper towel and set aside.

2. In a medium-sized pot, combine the milk, cheese wedges, mustard, spices, two teaspoons butter, and popcorn seasoning. Set heat to medium–low and stir the mixture frequently till melted and smooth.

3. Add the cornstarch and continue stirring till it thickens up. Remove from heat and add one cup of cheddar cheese and blend until melted. Adjust salt and pepper to taste (if mixture is too thick, add a teaspoon of almond milk).

4. Chop up the cauliflower into small chunks, then cut up the crêpe into vertical strips, then across horizontally in thirds, to resemble noodles.

5. Add the cauliflower chunks and the noodles to the cheese pot, and, with a large spoon, gently coat the cauliflower and noodles. Transfer to the prepared baking dish and smooth evenly across the top.

6. In a small bowl, combine the panko bread crumbs, parmesan, one-quarter cup cheddar cheese, and one teaspoon melted butter. Mix well and sprinkle evenly on top of the cauliflower.

Sides And Vegetables

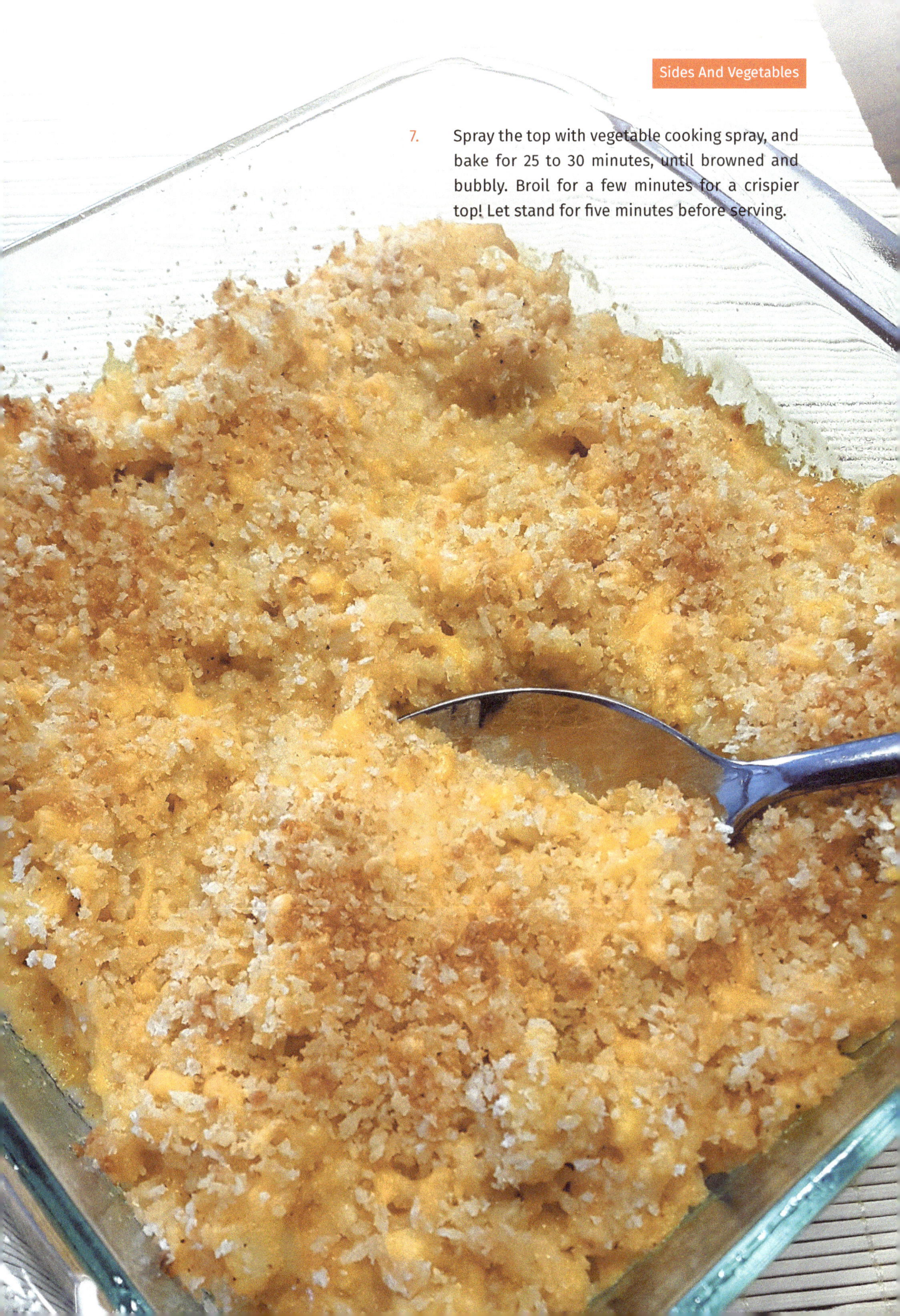

7. Spray the top with vegetable cooking spray, and bake for 25 to 30 minutes, until browned and bubbly. Broil for a few minutes for a crispier top! Let stand for five minutes before serving.

FAUX MASHED "POTATOES"

Cauliflower and a few ounces of white fleshed sweet potato are transformed into a comfort staple that allows us to keep on track while enjoying a tasty side vegetable without awakening the carb monster in us.

INGREDIENTS

½ medium cauliflower, washed and cut into large chunks

6 oz. white fleshed sweet potato, peeled and cut into chunks (cut a small portion from the large potato and store the rest in an opened plastic bag in the fridge)

1 T. butter

1 t. 0% plain Greek yogurt

½ t. garlic powder

½ t. onion powder

½ t. dried parsley

Salt and pepper to taste

INSTRUCTIONS

1. Fill a pot with salted water. Add cauliflower and sweet potato. Bring to a boil and continue a low boil until fork-tender (about 12 minutes). Remove from heat and drain in a colander in the sink. Allow to steam out as much moisture as possible. This may take about 10 minutes, but to guarantee a better texture, do not skip this step.

2. When you don't see any more steam, return the mixture to the original pot and add the spices, butter, and yogurt. Mash until smooth.

3. Adjust salt and pepper.

NOTE: If you find the texture still a bit wet, turn the heat on low and let more moisture evaporate. Stir frequently so it doesn't burn. As the mashed cauliflower cools down, it will continue to lose some wetness. Enjoy! I sometimes double the recipe, dividing it up into half-cup portions to freeze for single servings anytime, or to have on hand for other recipes.

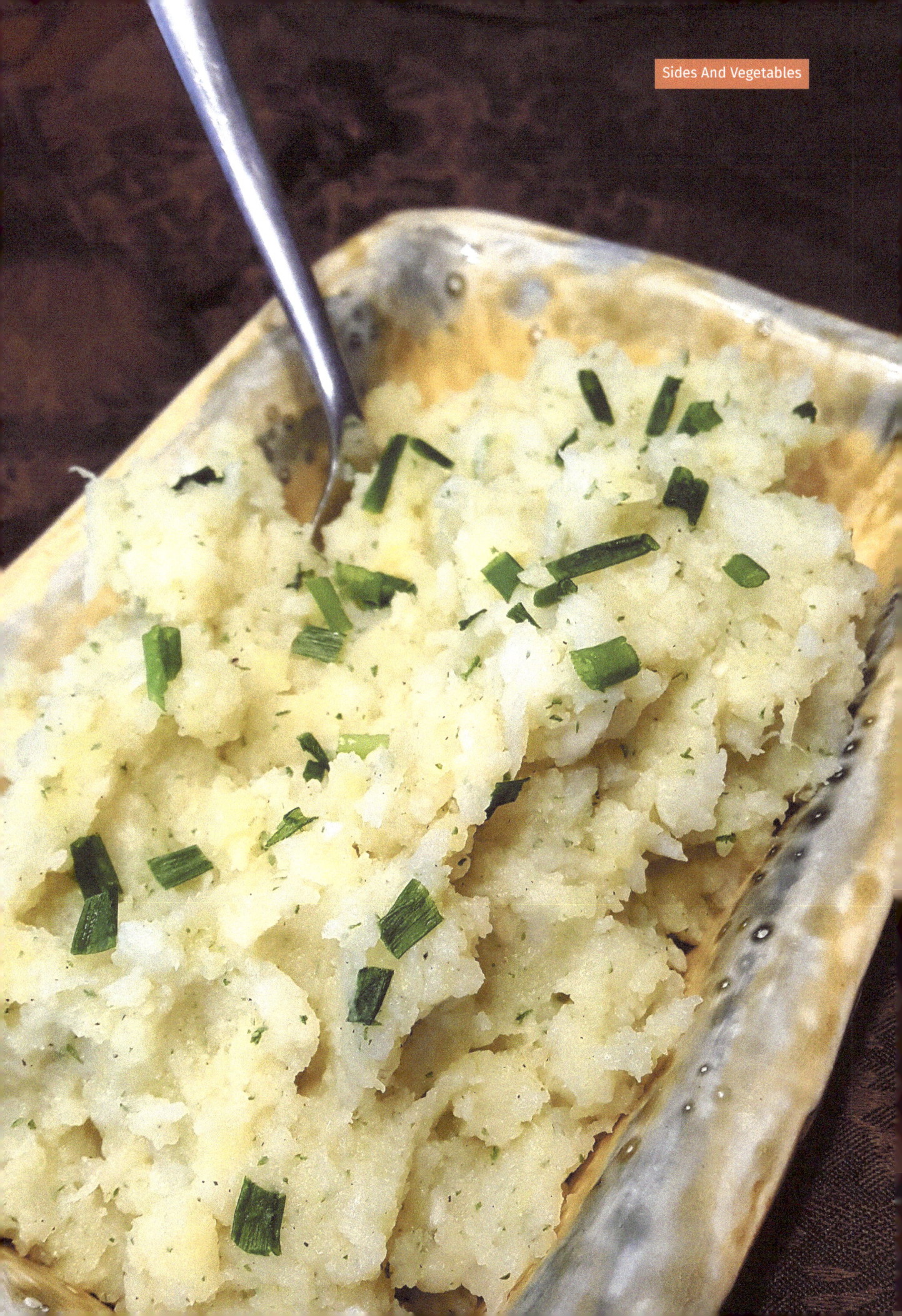

Sides And Vegetables

COMFORT COOKING
for Bariatric Post-Ops and Everyone Else!

TWICE-BAKED LOADED "POTATOES"

This is a great dish for buffet style entertaining because there are so many topping choices. Guests may help themselves to what they like!

INGREDIENTS

- 1 whole cauliflower, washed and cut into large chunks
- 10 oz. white fleshed sweet potato, cut into chunks
- 1 t. garlic powder
- 1 t. onion powder
- 1 t. sea salt
- ½ t. ground black pepper

- 2 T. butter
- 2 T. 0% plain Greek yogurt
- 4 oz. reduced-fat cheddar cheese, shredded
- 3 green onions, thinly sliced
- 1 T. dried parsley
- 1 T. dried onion flakes
- 2 eggs, beaten

INSTRUCTIONS

Pre-heat oven to 400°F and prepare a casserole dish with vegetable spray.

1. Boil cauliflower and sweet potato in salted water till fork-tender, about 12 minutes. Let steam out in a colander in the sink for about 10 minutes, or until you no longer see any steam. This step is of the utmost importance. The drier the better.

2. Return to pot then add all the remaining ingredients and mash until smooth. You may use your food processor; however, I find it a lot less work to just mash the old-fashioned way. Give the mixture a few good stirs with a wooden spoon.

3. Transfer to casserole dish and smooth the top evenly. Spray with vegetable spray then bake uncovered till puffed and golden, about 20 to 25 minutes. Turn on the broiler for the last few minutes to brown a bit more.

4. Serve with toppings: bacon bits, shredded reduced-fat cheddar, sliced green onions, plain Greek yogurt, or light sour cream.

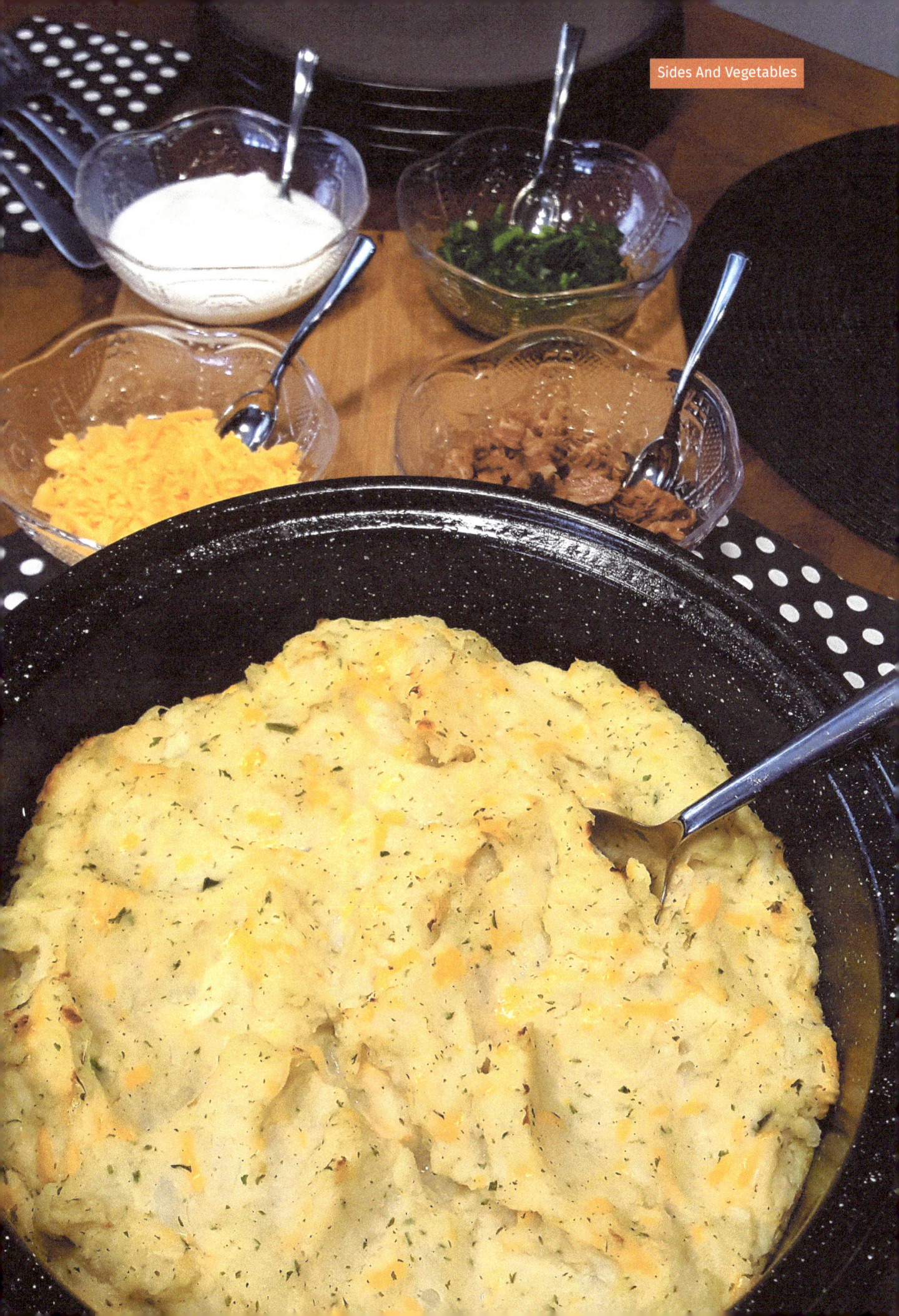

Sides And Vegetables

DELICIOUS OVEN-BAKED "TATER" TOTS

Oh yum! Make some of these as a side, or substitute for hash browns, or for an appetizer table and watch them disappear. Who knew that cauliflower would become THE magical stand-in for potatoes!

INGREDIENTS

Makes about 13 tots

- 2 c. cauliflower, (pulsed in food processor)
- 1 large egg, beaten
- 2 t. olive oil
- ½ c. onions, minced
- ¼ c. red pepper, minced
- ½ c. reduced fat cheddar cheese, shredded
- ¼ c. parmesan cheese
- ¼ c. panko bread crumbs
- ½ t. garlic powder
- ½ t. onion powder
- ¼ t. cayenne pepper
- 1 t. dried parsley flakes
- ¼ t. salt
- ¼ t. or more black pepper

INSTRUCTIONS

Pre-heat oven to 400°F and line a cookie sheet with parchment paper sprayed with vegetable spray.

1. Sauté riced cauliflower and onions in a non-stick skillet in olive oil over medium heat until softened. Add red pepper and continue to cook for two minutes longer. Set aside and allow to cool.
2. Transfer the cooled mixture to a medium-sized bowl and add all remaining ingredients. Mix well.
3. Using one heaping tablespoon of mixture at a time, shape into ovals using your hands and place them on the cookie sheet about one-half inch apart.
4. Spray the tots with vegetable spray, then bake for 20 minutes. Remove from oven and flip the tops and bake for five to 10 minutes longer, until golden and crispy.
5. Serve with no-sugar-added ketchup, salsa, Greek yogurt ranch dressing, or eat them plain!

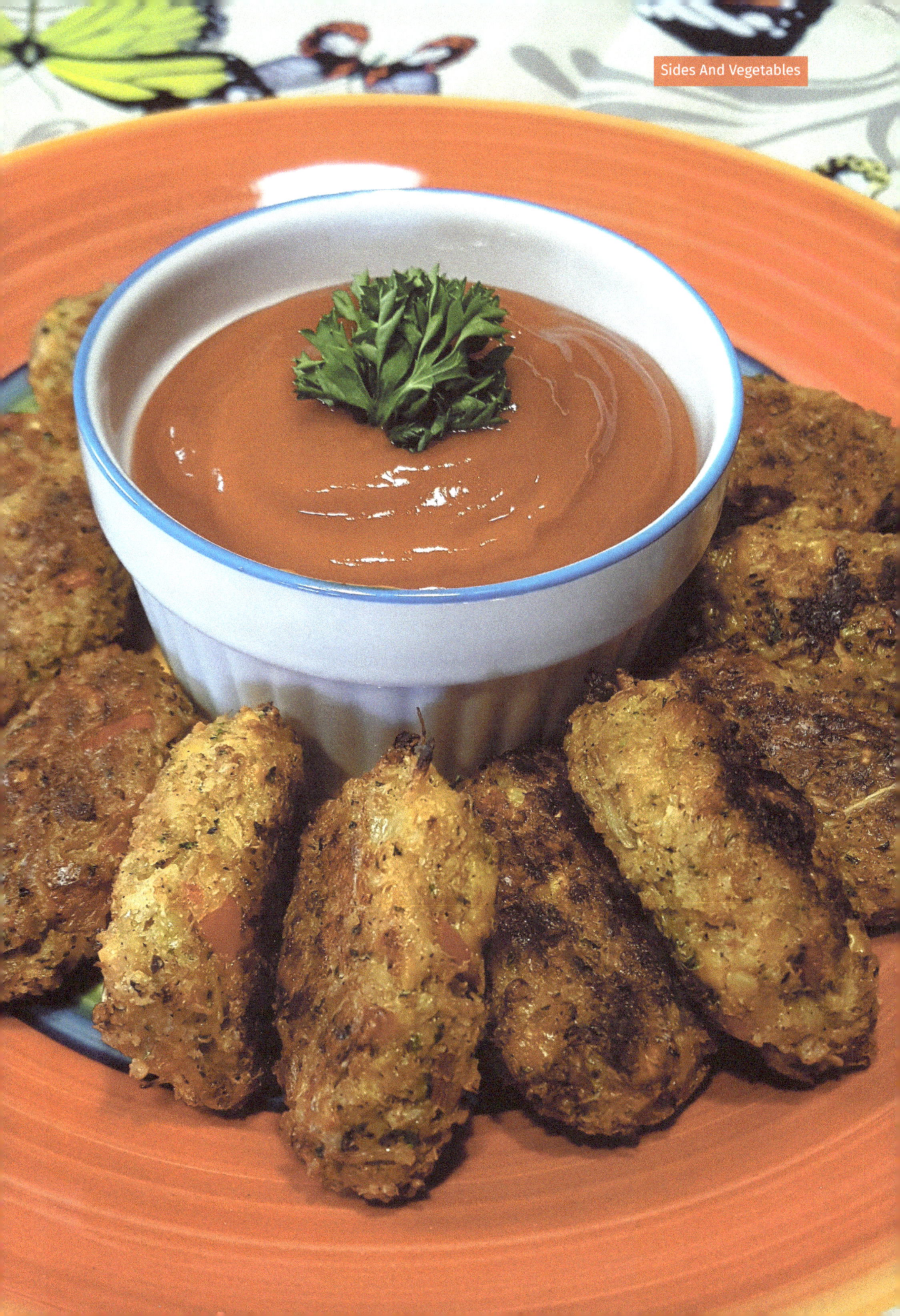

Sides And Vegetables

FRIED "RICE"

I am not a rice fan; however, when I make a stir fry or General Tso's Chicken, it does not seem complete without the "rice." This one's a winner!

INGREDIENTS

1 t. sesame oil

1 t. ginger, grated

2 garlic cloves, minced

¼ c. onion, chopped

¼ c. carrot, shredded

1 T. green peas, thawed

½ head cauliflower, about 5 c. (pulse in food processor)

3 T. soy sauce or less

1 T. Truvia Brown Sugar Blend

1 t. sesame oil, added at the end

3 green onions, thinly sliced

½ t. chili flakes

Salt and pepper to taste

1 egg, beaten

INSTRUCTIONS

1. Using a non-stick skillet over high heat, add the sesame oil, ginger, garlic, onion, carrot, and peas. Cook for three minutes. Add cauliflower and continue to cook for another three minutes, until softened.
2. Add soy sauce, Truvia, green onions, and chili flakes. Mix well.
3. Add the beaten egg, and stir until the egg becomes cooked and distributed.
4. Remove from heat and stir in one teaspoon sesame oil.
5. Taste and adjust with more soy sauce and pepper, if needed.

NOTE: If you want plain "rice" as a side dish without the Asian flavours, follow the recipe but omit the ginger, Truvia, soy sauce, and sesame oil. Use olive oil instead. For a Spanish "rice," add two tablespoons of tomato paste to the skillet. If you want a traditional light-coloured fried rice, go easy on the soy sauce.

Sides And Vegetables

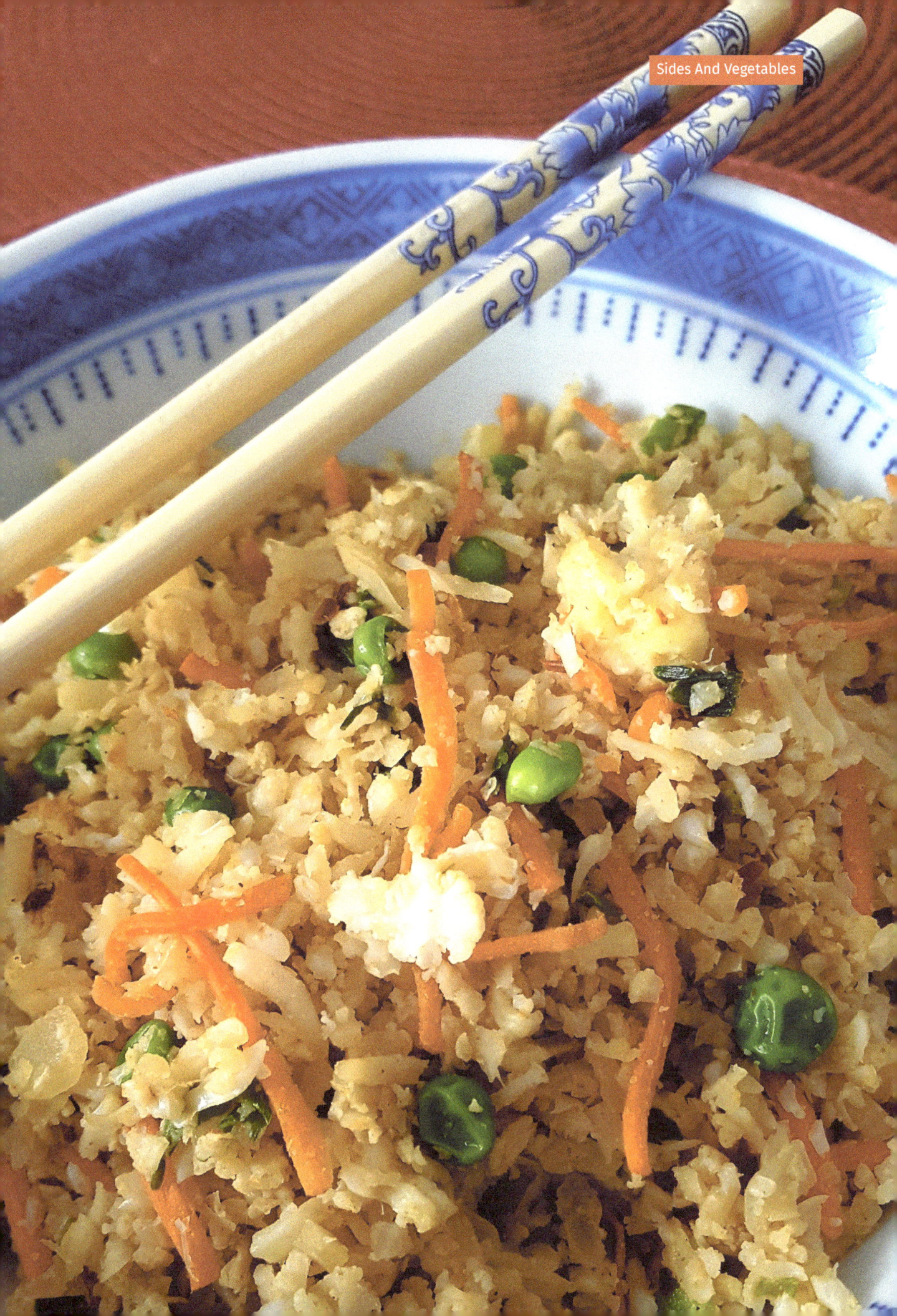

LOW-CARB "FLATBREAD" (BECAUSE SOMETIMES YOU JUST NEED TO MAKE A SANDWICH)

For the occasional time when you just don't feel like sandwiching between two lettuce leaves. These resemble pancakes but are savory without a lot of nasty carbs. They are really good as is or toasted. Not eggy at all. This recipe makes eight ovals. Each flatbread has approximately six carbs. Use only half of one for only three carbs. Make a half sandwich and pair it with a hot bowl of soup.

INGREDIENTS

- 2 eggs
- 1 t. olive oil
- ½ c. milk (I use ¼ c. unsweetened almond milk and ¼ c. 1% milk)
- ¼ t. of salt
- Dash of ground black pepper
- ½ c. baking mix (I use Bisquick original)
- 1 t. parmesan cheese
- ½ t. dried Italian seasoning
- ¼ t. garlic powder
- ¼ t. onion powder
- 1½ t. baking powder

INSTRUCTIONS

1. In a medium-sized bowl, whisk wet ingredients until smooth. In another bowl, mix dry ingredients and blend well.
2. Add the dry to the wet in three batches, mixing after each addition till smooth (no lumps).
3. Spray a skillet with vegetable spray and heat up to medium. Using a tad less than one-quarter cup at a time, pour batter into skillet in a small round (holding the skillet handle, angle the skillet to spread the batter out in an oval shape) and watch for flatbread to dry at the edges and form tiny holes (about one minute or less).
4. Flip gently and cook for about 30 seconds. Place on a wire rack to cool. Continue until batter is finished.
5. Store them in the freezer, in between wax paper, and use as needed.

NOTE: Thaw and cut in half and use as you would two slices of bread. You can toast them for a bit of crispness or just fold in half as is. Fill with ham or turkey, cheese, tomatoes, onions, etc., half-fat mayonnaise and mustard. Yum! OR make an awesome grilled cheese by cutting one flatbread in half and grilling in a skillet. Make sure you use reduced-fat cheese!

Sides And Vegetables

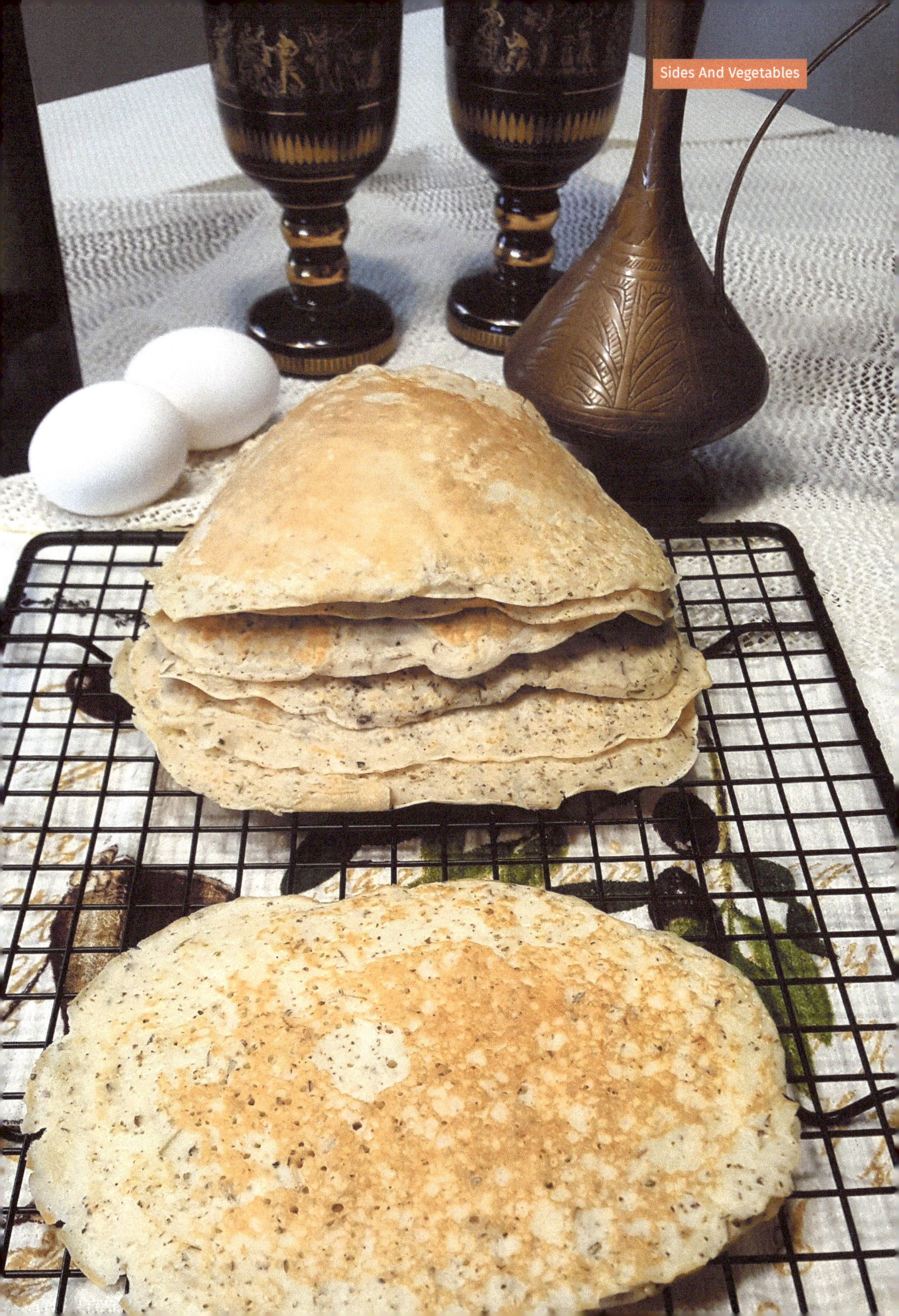

LOW-CARB CRÊPES (PASTA SUBSTITUTE)

These are incredibly versatile. I make several batches at one time and store them in the freezer between wax paper. I use them for all my "pasta" needs.

INGREDIENTS

Makes nine or ten crêpes

- ⅔ c. flour
- ½ t. salt
- 2 eggs
- ¾ c. milk (I use ½ c. unsweetened almond milk plus ¼ c. 1% milk)
- 1 T. olive oil

INSTRUCTIONS

1. Whisk wet ingredients together, then add dry ingredients and whisk until smooth (no lumps).
2. Cover with plastic wrap and refrigerate for one hour.
3. Remove from fridge. Batter should be thin. If you feel it's a bit thick, thin out with a little water, one teaspoon at a time.
4. Spray an 8-inch, non-stick skillet with vegetable spray and heat on medium–high heat. Using a little less than one-quarter cup at a time, coat the skillet by tilting the pan to quickly distribute the batter in a round.
5. Lower the heat to medium–low and let the crêpe cook for about two minutes. Loosen the edges with a spatula, and flip to cook a minute longer. Transfer to a plate and repeat with the remaining batter, spraying the skillet as needed.

NOTE A: I use this "pasta" substitute for noodles and layered casseroles, etc. To cut into noodle form, cut strips vertically (thin or thick), then horizontally in thirds. Use them in recipes as suggested. To use as "pasta" layers, simply place a crêpe on top of your filling and repeat as needed. If you don't like the gaps of the top layer, cut an extra crêpe up to fill them in.

NOTE B: These crêpes are extremely thin and are not rubbery like pasta so you should have no problem eating them. They should never result in a "stuck" episode. Remember that each crêpe has about three carbs each and you are not eating six of them all at once. For me, in order for a recipe to match up to the real thing, I need the right texture, taste, and visual to convince my taste-buds and brain. This is it and this is why these "pasta" look-alikes are so important to my recipes.

Sides And Vegetables

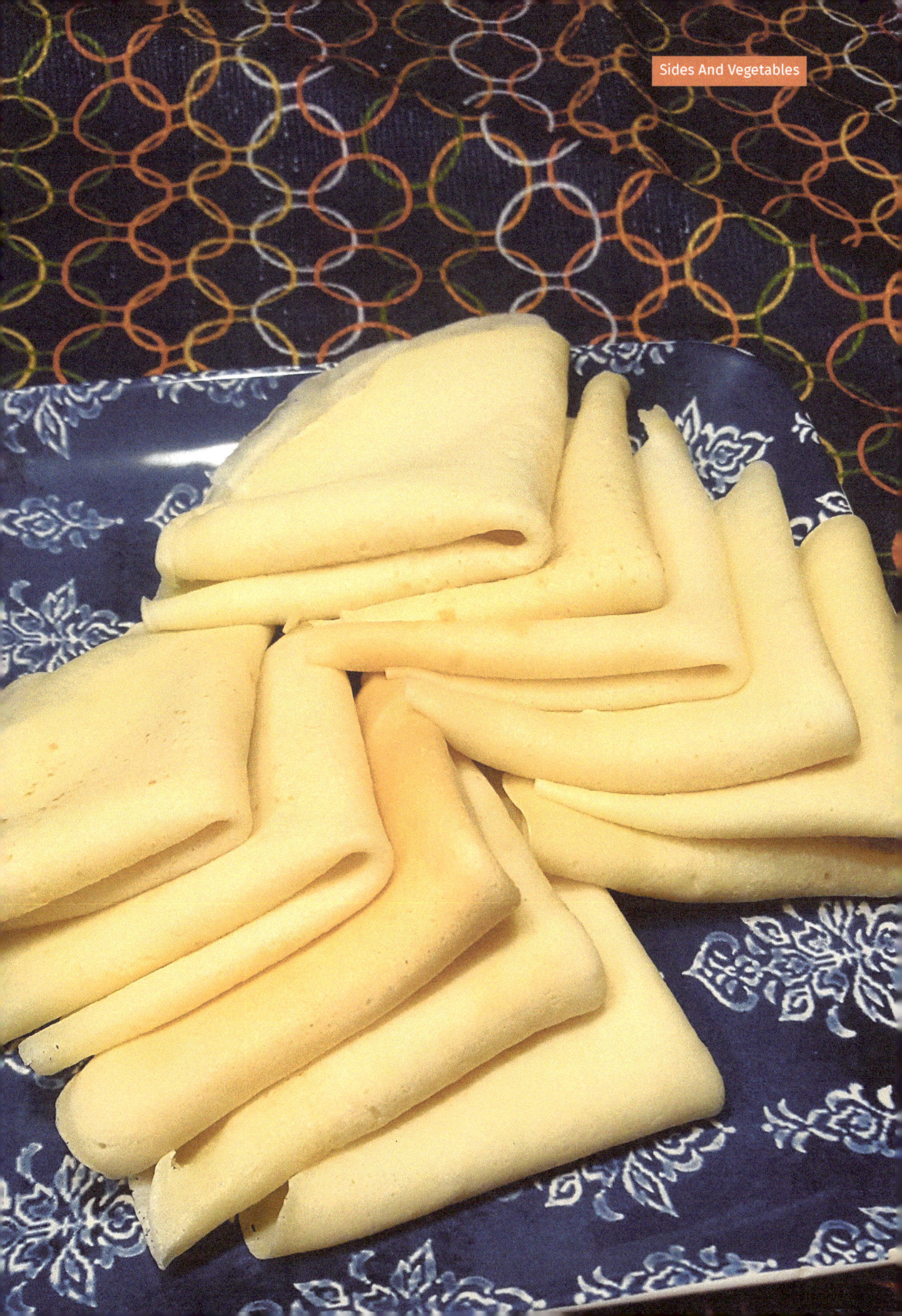

COMFORT COOKING
for Bariatric Post-Ops and Everyone Else!

FRIED CABBAGE WITH ONIONS AND "PASTA" SQUARES

Another one of my mom's fabulous Hungarian recipes made easy, delicious, AND bariatric-friendly. Once again, the "pasta" crêpe provides the right texture, visual appeal, and taste to the dish.

INGREDIENTS

- 2 T. olive oil plus 1 t. butter
- 1 medium onion, chopped
- ½ medium head cabbage, cored and chopped into squares
- Ground black pepper to taste
- Salt to taste
- 1 Low-Carb Crêpe (recipe found on previous page), cut into squares

INSTRUCTIONS

1. In a large skillet, sauté cabbage and onions in olive oil and butter until golden brown and tender, about 25 minutes. Season with salt and black pepper.
2. Gently add the "pasta" squares to the skillet and carefully distribute. Give it one last taste for salt and pepper and adjust accordingly. Rewarm to serve piping hot.

NOTE: To cut crêpe into squares, simply cut vertically into strips, then horizontally across to form small squares.

Sides And Vegetables

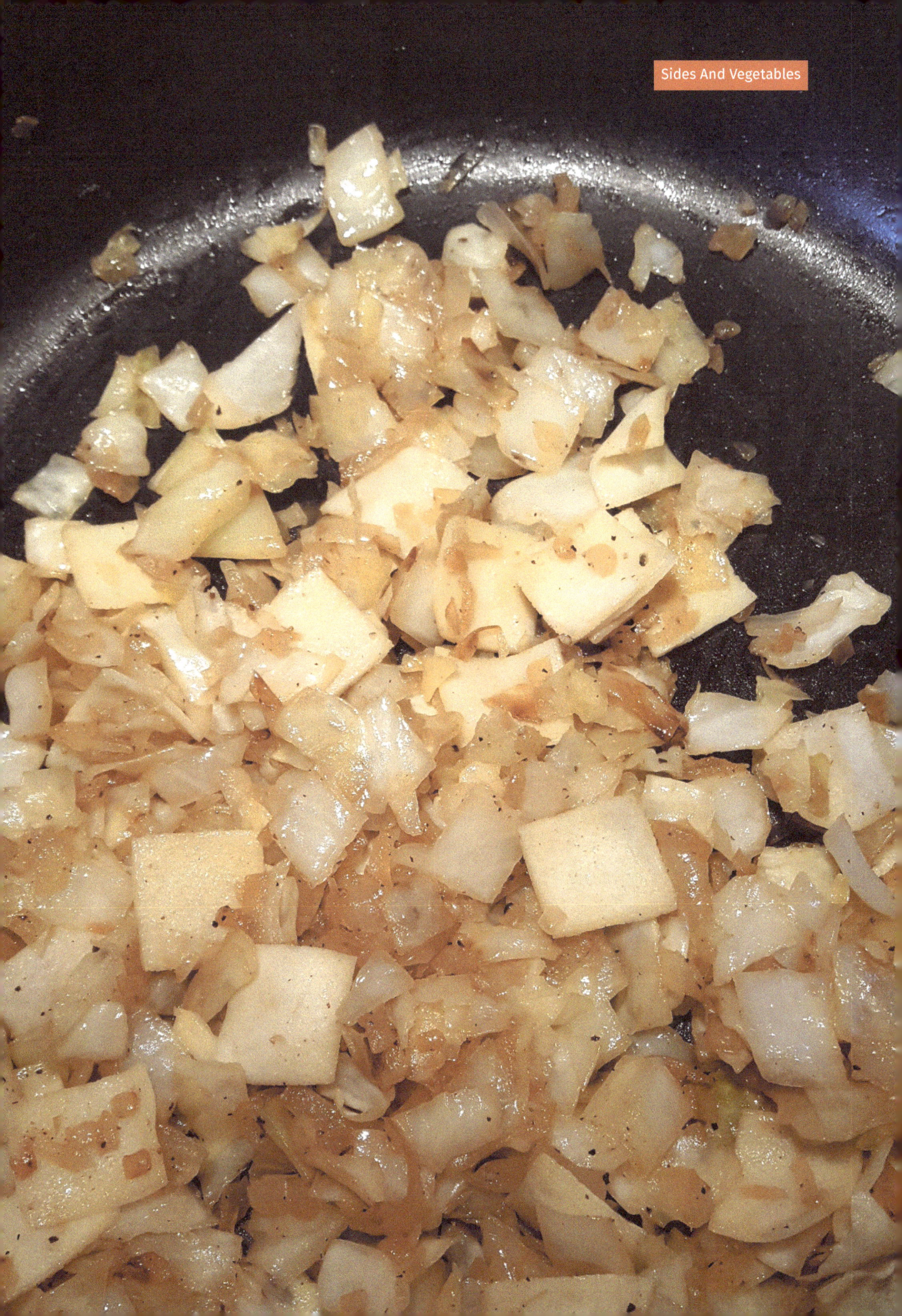

HOLIDAY STUFFING

Who doesn't love stuffing! This is a healthier version, with much less bread than the traditional kind. It is perfect for the holiday table or for a special-occasion dinner. This is not something that you would be eating frequently, so do not obsess about the "stuffing cubes." Have a few tablespoons and let your guests enjoy the rest!

INGREDIENTS

1 lb. Italian sausage

2 c. celery, diced finely

2 c. onions, diced finely

2 c. Granny Smith apples, diced finely

2 T. butter

2 T. olive oil

1 T. garlic powder

2 t. salt

1 t. black pepper

1 t. dried thyme

2 T. poultry seasoning

3 c. bread stuffing cubes

1 egg, beaten

2 T. dried parsley

Low-sodium chicken broth

INSTRUCTIONS

1. Brown sausage in a large skillet. Add celery, onions, apples, butter, and olive oil, and cook over medium-high heat, until onions are softened. Stir in all spices.

2. Place the bread cubes into a separate large bowl. Add the sausage mixture and toss to combine. Add the egg and a little chicken broth, just enough to make a moist stuffing.

3. You can stuff your turkey or chicken with this stuffing and bake accordingly or transfer stuffing into an oven dish sprayed with vegetable spray, cover with foil and bake for 20 minutes at 350°F, then uncover, spray the top, and bake an additional 20 minutes, until golden brown. Broil for a few minutes, if necessary.

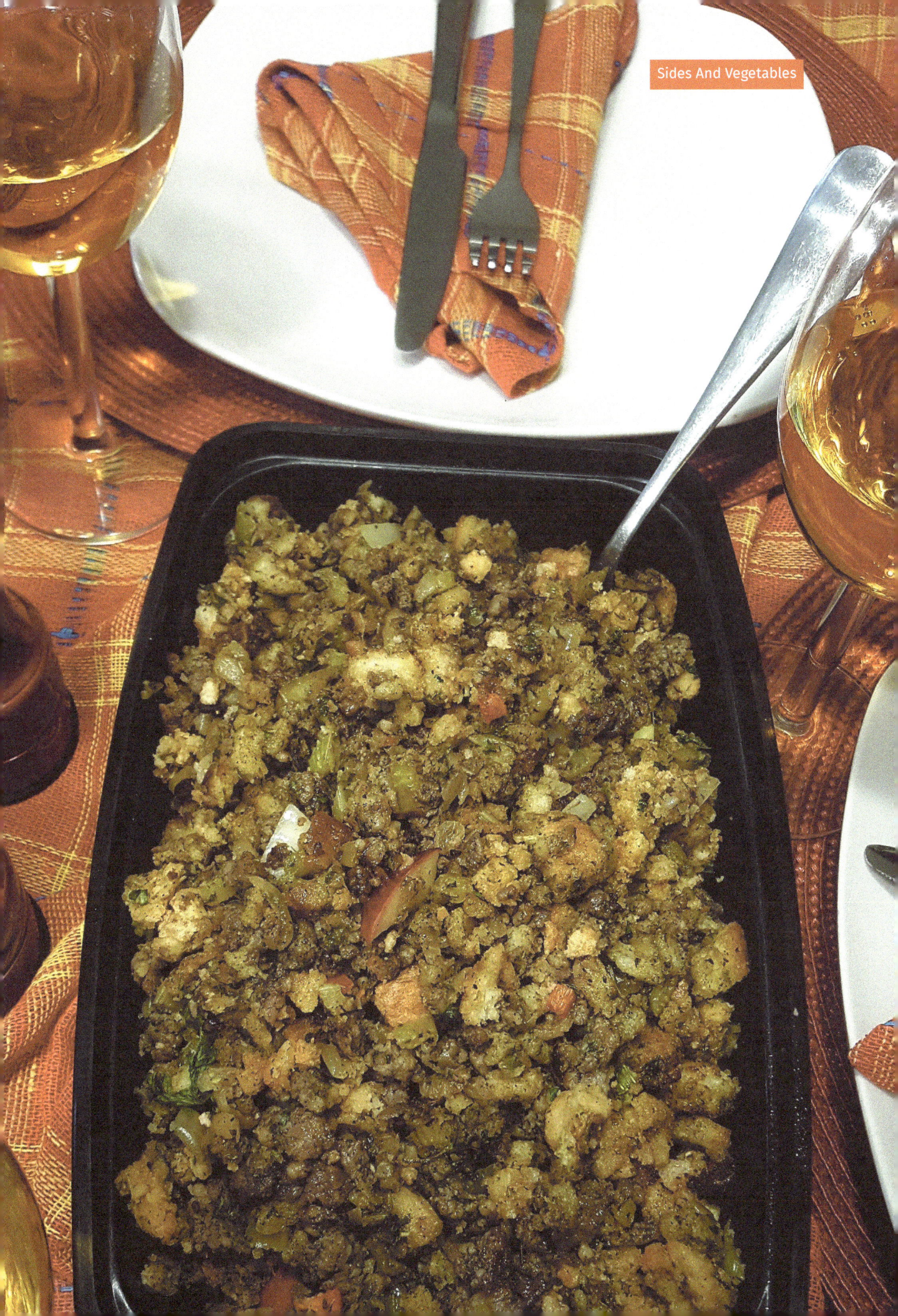

Sides And Vegetables

CHEESE LATKES

Oy! Are these ever good! Latkes usually make a yearly appearance during Chanukah, but thanks to this recipe, they are not just for holidays anymore. These golden nuggets are full of protein, low in carbs, and taste almost identical to the potato kind! Enjoy them any time or even as a light lunch paired with a salad.

INGREDIENTS

½ medium onion, minced

1 T. butter

1 t. olive oil

Salt and ground black pepper to taste

1 c. reduced-fat ricotta cheese

2 eggs, beaten

3 T. flour

Vegetable cooking spray

INSTRUCTIONS

1. In a non-stick skillet, sauté onions in butter and olive oil until nicely browned. Add salt and black pepper to taste. Remove from heat and transfer to a small plate to cool.

2. In a small bowl, whisk together cheese, eggs, and flour, until smooth. Add cooled onions and stir to combine.

3. Spray the same skillet with vegetable spray, heat up to medium and drop about two tablespoons of batter at a time to form small pancakes. Make sure to leave enough room so they do not touch. Cook about two minutes per side then transfer to a warming plate or place into a 200°F oven to keep warm until ready to serve. Continue cooking the pancakes in small batches, until batter is gone.

4. Serve warm, topped with 0% plain Greek yogurt or light sour cream and thinly sliced green onion.

NOTE: If you have a large crowd at home, make sure to double the recipe! There will not be any leftovers.

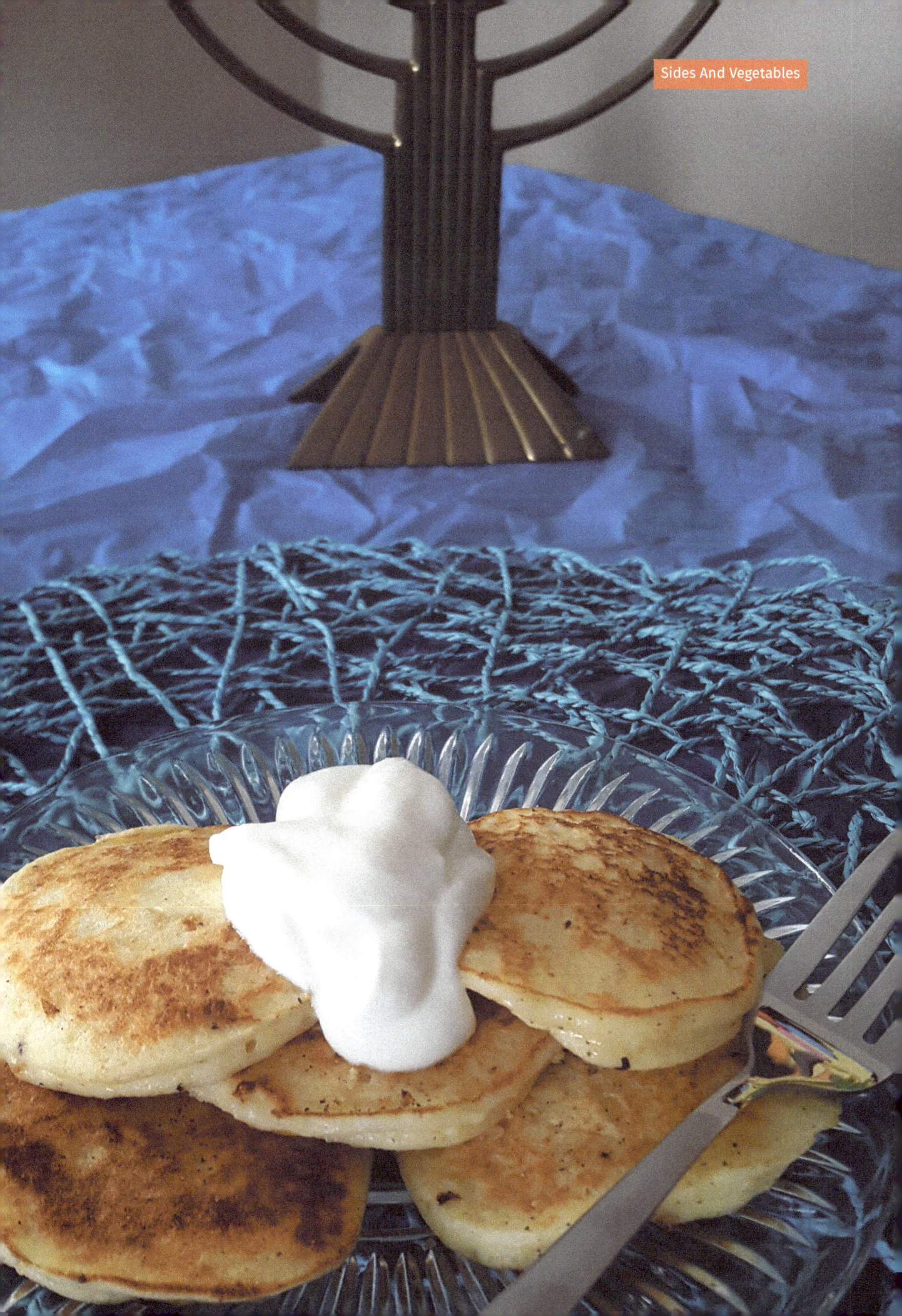

Sides And Vegetables

COMFORT COOKING
for Bariatric Post-Ops and Everyone Else!

LAZY PEROGY CASSEROLE

Being from Winnipeg, perogies have always been a big deal to me. What lies below is nothing other than pure genius. For all of you perogy lovers and for all of you future fans, I give you my very best! You will be weeping tears of joy after your first bite.

INGREDIENTS

1 lb. white flesh sweet potato, peeled and cubed

½ medium head cauliflower, cut into large florets

1 large onion, chopped

2 t. olive oil

1 T. butter

Salt and ground black pepper to taste (I use a lot of black pepper)

1 c. reduced-fat cheddar cheese, shredded

2 t. onion powder

1 T. 0% plain Greek yogurt

¼ c. cooked bacon, crumbled (optional, but yummy)

More salt

3 Low-Carb Crêpes (recipe found in Sides)

INSTRUCTIONS

1. In a large skillet, sauté the onions in olive oil and butter, until lightly browned. Add salt and ground black pepper to taste. Set aside.

2. In a large pot, boil cauliflower and sweet potato in salted water for about 12 minutes, until softened. Drain into a colander in the sink and allow to steam out for 10 minutes or until you do not see any steam. This is VERY important. If left too wet, then the mixture will be mushy.

3. Return to pot and add the browned onions, cheese, onion powder, yogurt, and bacon. Mash all the goodness until smooth and well combined. If mixture is too stiff, add a bit more yogurt until it reaches the proper consistency. Not too loose, but not too stiff. Taste, and add more salt. Because sweet potatoes are much sweeter than regular potatoes, they require a bit more salt to mask the sweetness. Add a bit more pepper, too; it can't hurt. Set aside.

4. Spray an 8 × 8 glass baking dish with vegetable spray. Begin with one crêpe on the bottom. Add one-half of the filling over the bottom crêpe and smooth out evenly. Cover with the second crêpe. Add the other half of the filling and smooth it out evenly. Place the third crêpe over top. If you like, take an extra crêpe out and cut strips to fill in the gaps on the top.

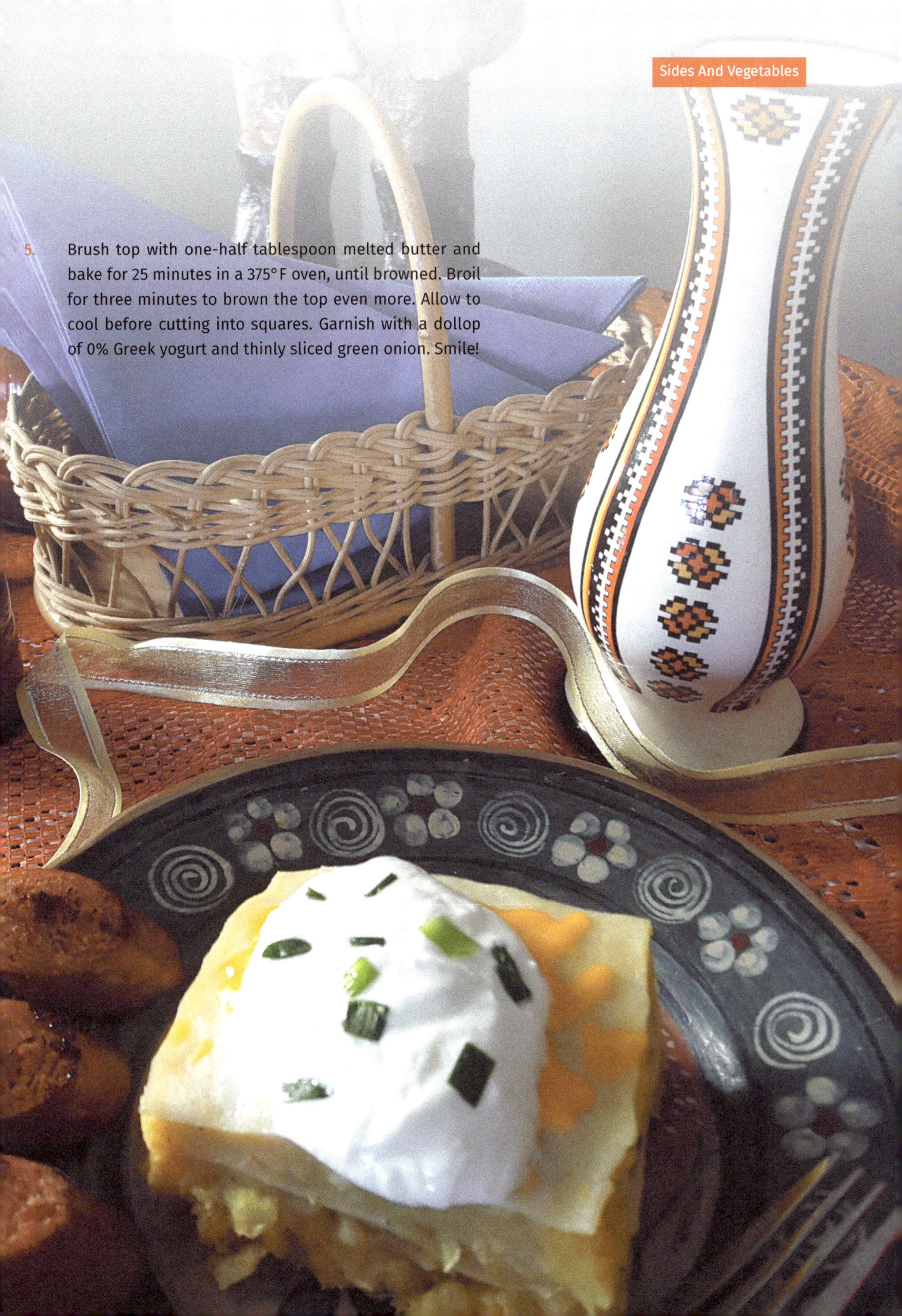

Sides And Vegetables

5. Brush top with one-half tablespoon melted butter and bake for 25 minutes in a 375°F oven, until browned. Broil for three minutes to brown the top even more. Allow to cool before cutting into squares. Garnish with a dollop of 0% Greek yogurt and thinly sliced green onion. Smile!

ROASTED GARLICKY BRUSSEL SPROUTS

I was never a fan of Brussel sprouts until I perfected this recipe. Be ready to call it your new favourite!

INGREDIENTS

15 Brussel sprouts, halved (use fresh, otherwise the texture will be off)

1 T. butter

1 T. olive oil

3 cloves garlic, smashed

Salt and pepper to taste

2 T. crisp bacon, crumbled (optional, but yummy)

INSTRUCTIONS

1. Melt butter and olive oil in a large skillet over medium-high heat. When butter is foamy, reduce heat to medium-low and add garlic, then cook until lightly browned, about three to five minutes.

2. With a slotted spoon, remove the garlic and discard. Add Brussel sprouts, cut-side down. Sprinkle a pinch of sea salt over them, then cover and cook on medium-low heat for about 12 to 15 minutes. Do not stir. Sprouts should be fork-tender after 15 minutes.

3. Gently turn Brussel sprouts over with a fork. Add the bacon, salt if necessary, and pepper to taste.

4. Carefully coat and distribute all the goodness evenly. Plate and enjoy paired with a protein dish.

Sides And Vegetables

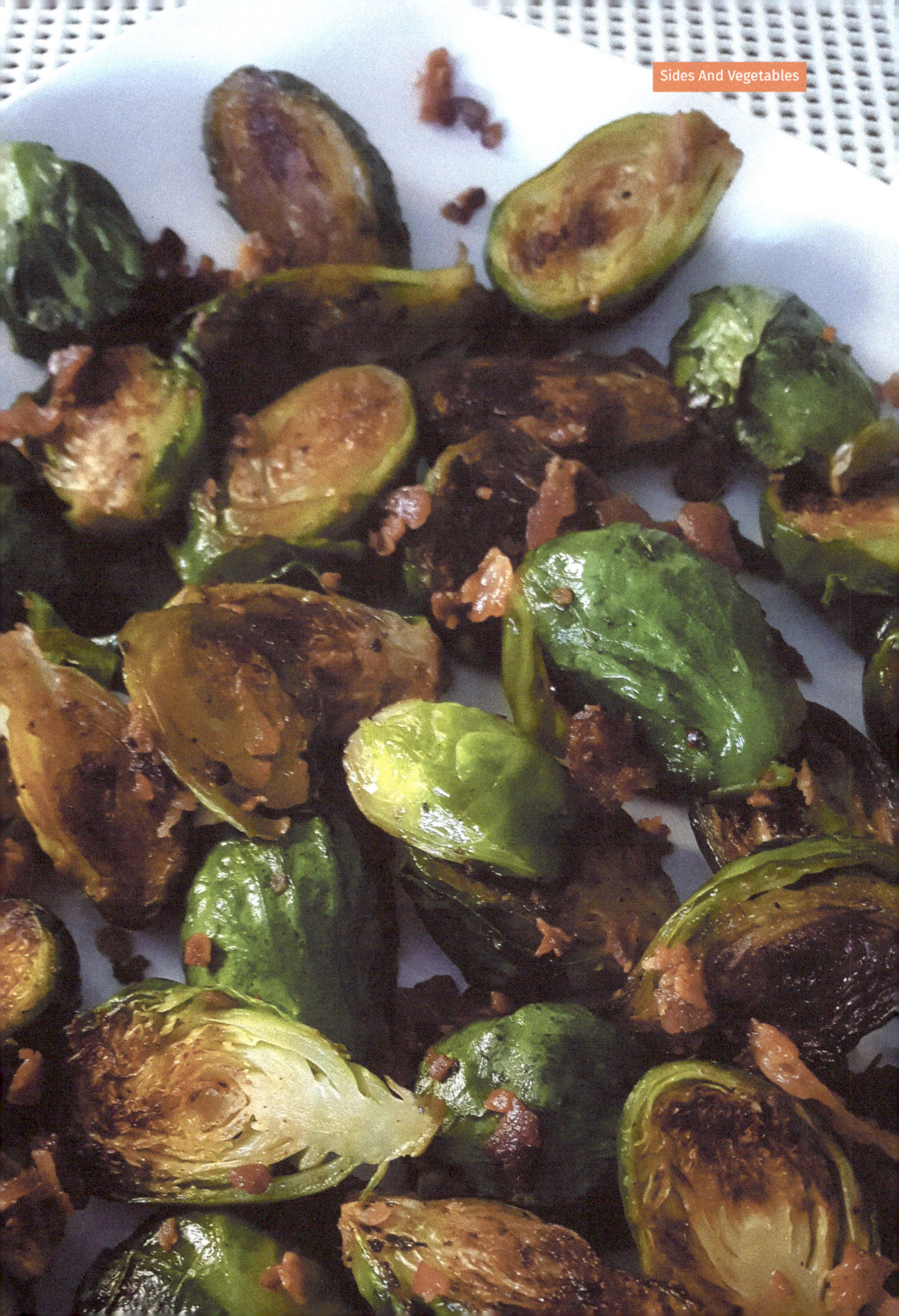

COMFORT COOKING
for Bariatric Post-Ops and Everyone Else!

BREAD AND BUTTER PICKLES

I just love a few of these with a portion of my Chili Mac Skillet (page 90) or with a slice of Cheeseburger Pie (page 72).

INGREDIENTS

1 c. jarred sliced hamburger pickles (I use Bick's hamburger slices)

3 T. Truvia Baking Blend

1 T. white vinegar

1 t. yellow mustard

Pinch of salt and pepper to taste

INSTRUCTIONS

1. Lightly rinse the pickles once in cold water, drain slightly, but keep them wet, and transfer to a bowl.
2. Combine pickles with white Truvia, vinegar, and mustard, then add a pinch of salt and ground black pepper to taste.
3. Mix well. Place pickles in a small mason jar and pour the liquid over the pickles.
4. Store in the fridge and, each time you take some out of the jar, make sure to give the jar a shake to coat the pickles with the brine.

NOTE: If you feel you need them sweeter, feel free to adjust the amount of Truvia. You could easily double the recipe as your family will enjoy them, too!

Sides And Vegetables

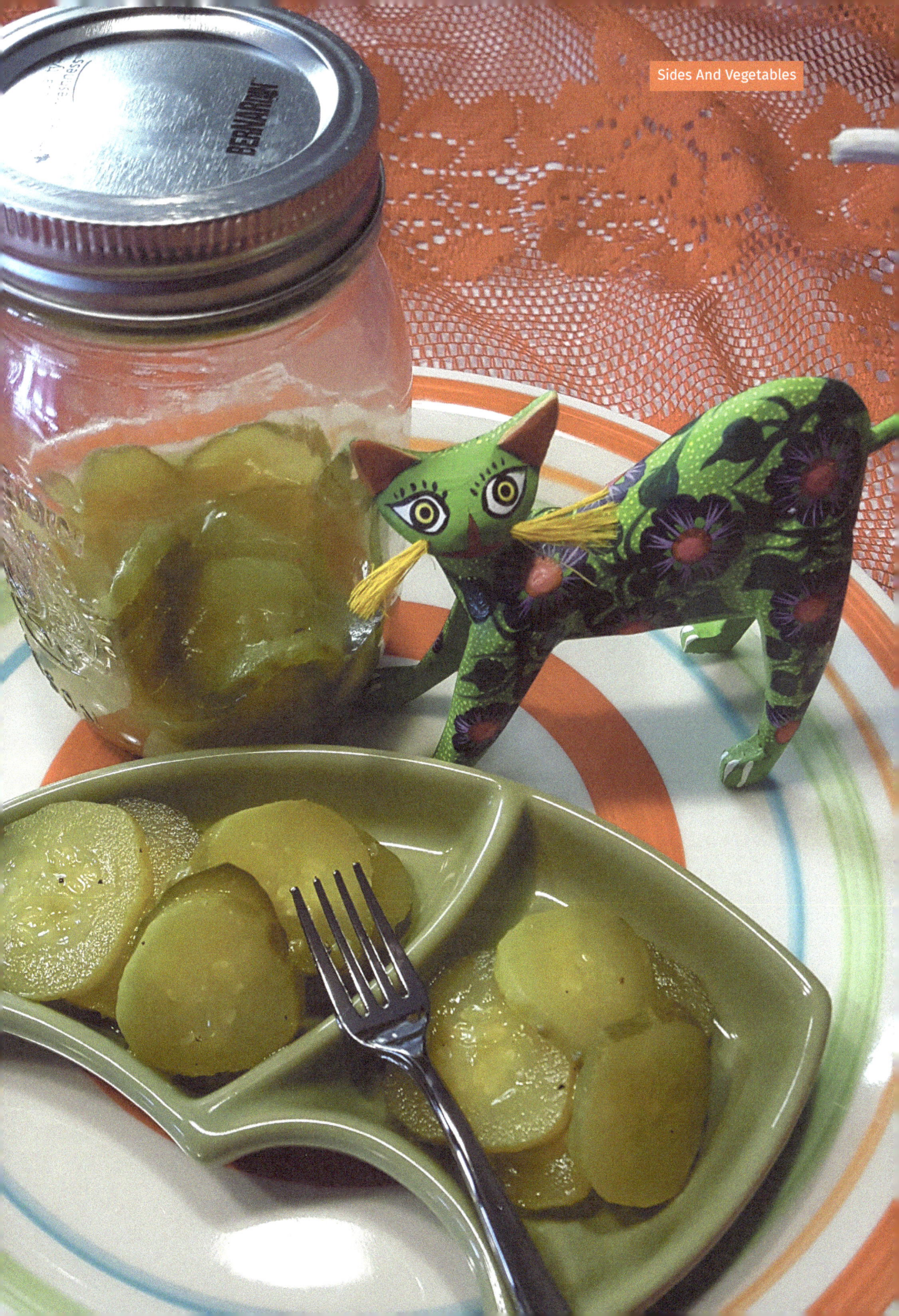

COMFORT COOKING
for Bariatric Post-Ops and Everyone Else!

GREEN BEAN CASSEROLE MAKEOVER

How do you spell comfort? G-r-e-e-n-b-e-a-n-c-a-s-s-e-r-o-l-e-m-a-k-e-o-v-e-r. This is a delicious dish for the holiday table or a special dinner gathering. The crispy dehydrated onion bits make this dish worth the effort. This will become YOUR celebration signature dish!

INGREDIENTS

- 1 lb. fresh green beans
- 8 oz. mushrooms, sliced
- ½ c. onions, sliced
- 3 cloves garlic, minced
- 2 T. butter
- 1 t. salt
- ½ t. ground black pepper
- ½ t. paprika
- ½ t. garlic powder
- ¼ t. ground nutmeg
- 2 T. white flour
- 1 c. low-sodium chicken broth
- 1 c. 1% milk
- ½ c. reduced-fat cheddar cheese, shredded
- 2 T. dried dehydrated onion (find this in the spice section of your store)

INSTRUCTIONS

1. In a medium-sized pot, boil the beans in salted water until tender, about 10 to 15 minutes. Drain then set aside.

2. Melt butter in a large skillet over medium–high heat, until it starts to foam. Add onions, reduce heat to medium–low, then cook onions until browned and tender, about 15 minutes.

3. Add mushrooms and garlic and continue cooking until mushrooms are partly dry. Add the pepper, paprika, garlic powder, and nutmeg, and mix until well combined.

4. Sprinkle flour over the mixture and cook for one minute. Add broth and milk and cook for three to five minutes, stirring frequently, until it starts to thicken and bubble.

5. Remove from heat and gently fold in green beans and cheese. Transfer mixture into a casserole dish sprayed with vegetable spray. Add the dehydrated onion to the same skillet, turn the heat up to medium and stir up all the bits with the onion as it browns. Remove from heat and sprinkle the onion on top of the casserole. Spray the top with vegetable spray and bake, uncovered, at 350°F for 15 minutes. Serve hot!

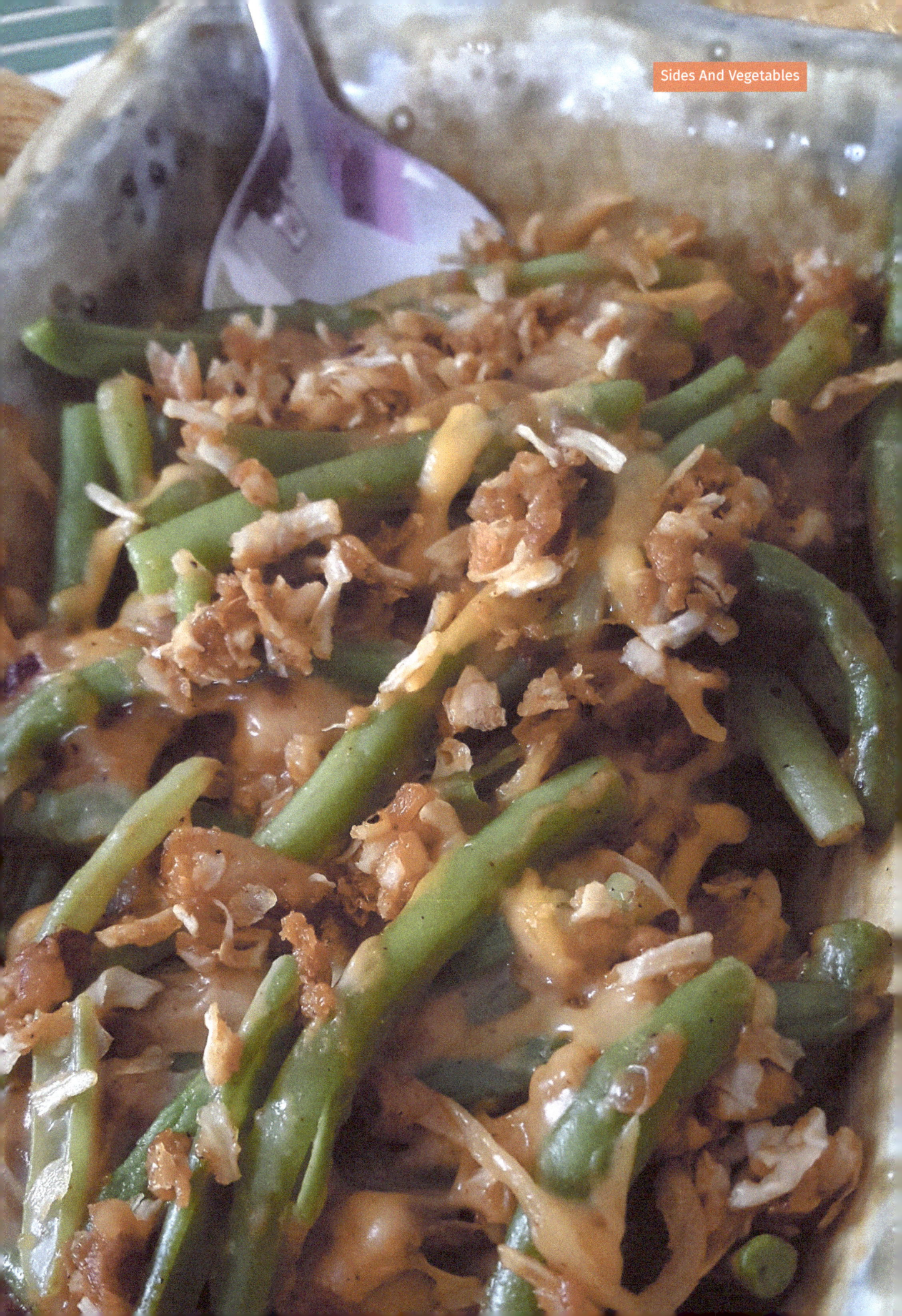

Sides And Vegetables

SPIRAL VEGGIE "NOODLES"

The vegetable spiralizer is a game-changer for those who adore pasta but have drawn a hard line of striking it off the food list. If you do not have one, get one as soon as possible and you will not know how you lived without it. I use the "Veggetti."

INGREDIENTS

Zucchini noodles—that's it!

INSTRUCTIONS

1. Sauté zucchini in a little olive oil and minced garlic just for a minute or two, otherwise it will become mushy.
2. Top with your favourite sauce and add a protein. It doesn't get any easier than that!

NOTE: Spaghetti squash is another way to have your noodles and eat it. Slice the squash into one and one-half-inch slices, remove the seeds, place in a single layer on a cookie sheet, drizzle with a little olive oil, and sprinkle with a pinch of sea salt, then roast in a 400°F oven for 30 minutes or so. Pierce skin with a knife to test for readiness. Using a fork, scrape the squash out by pulling the flesh from the peel to separate the strands. Serve immediately with your favourite sauce!

Sides And Vegetables

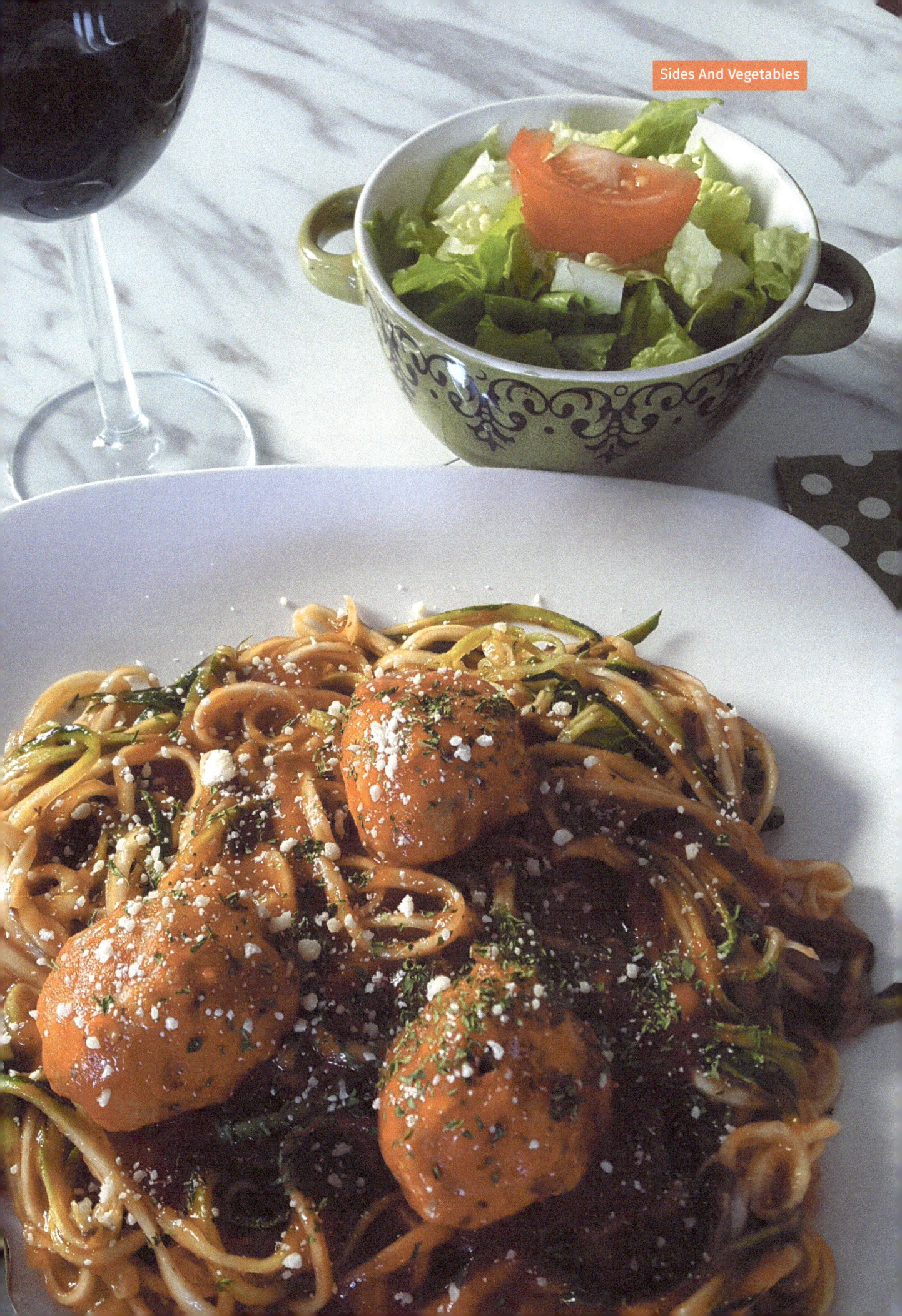

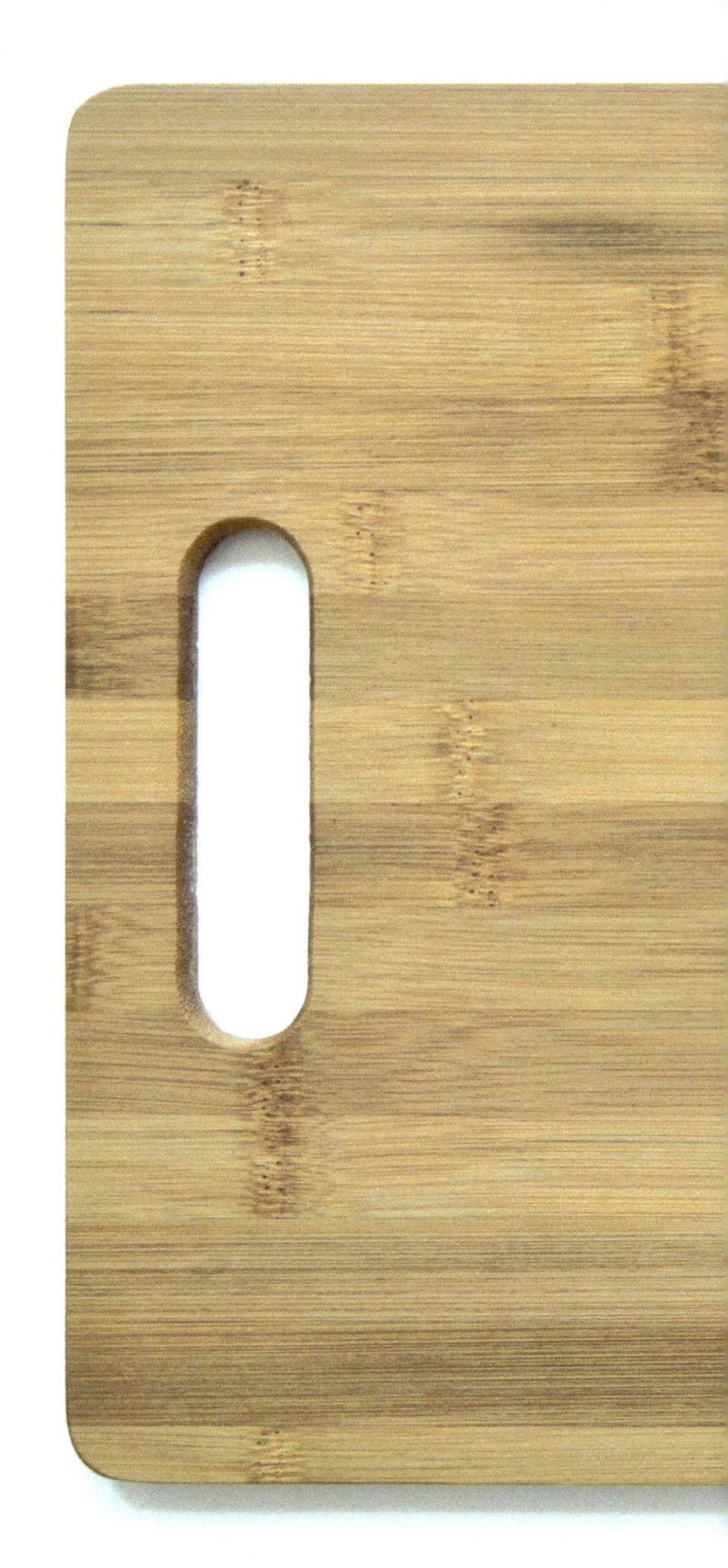

GRAVY AND SAUCES

Mushroom Gravy 150

Chicken Gravy 152

No-Sugar BBQ Sauce 154

Blueberry Sauce 156

Chocolate Dipping Sauce 158

COMFORT COOKING
for Bariatric Post-Ops and Everyone Else!

MUSHROOM GRAVY

Simple to prepare, this gravy is a staple in our house. Spooned over meats or Faux Mashed "Potatoes," it is comfort gravy at its best!

INGREDIENTS

½ c. low-sodium beef broth

½ c. water

1 package brown or mushroom gravy mix (I use Clubhouse)

3 oz. white mushrooms, sliced

1 t. butter

½ c. low-fat milk

Ground black pepper to taste

INSTRUCTIONS

1. In a medium-sized skillet, melt butter over medium heat. Add mushrooms and sauté until browned and tender, about four minutes. Transfer the mushrooms into a small bowl.

2. In another small bowl, dissolve the gravy mix into the beef broth using a whisk. Add the water and then the milk, stirring well to combine. Add the liquid to the skillet and set the heat back to medium-high while whisking the gravy until it boils and thickens, about two minutes.

3. Return the mushrooms to the skillet and blend well. Remove from heat and add pepper to taste.

4. Enjoy!

NOTE: You can use pan drippings, if available, in place of the beef broth.

Gravy And Sauces

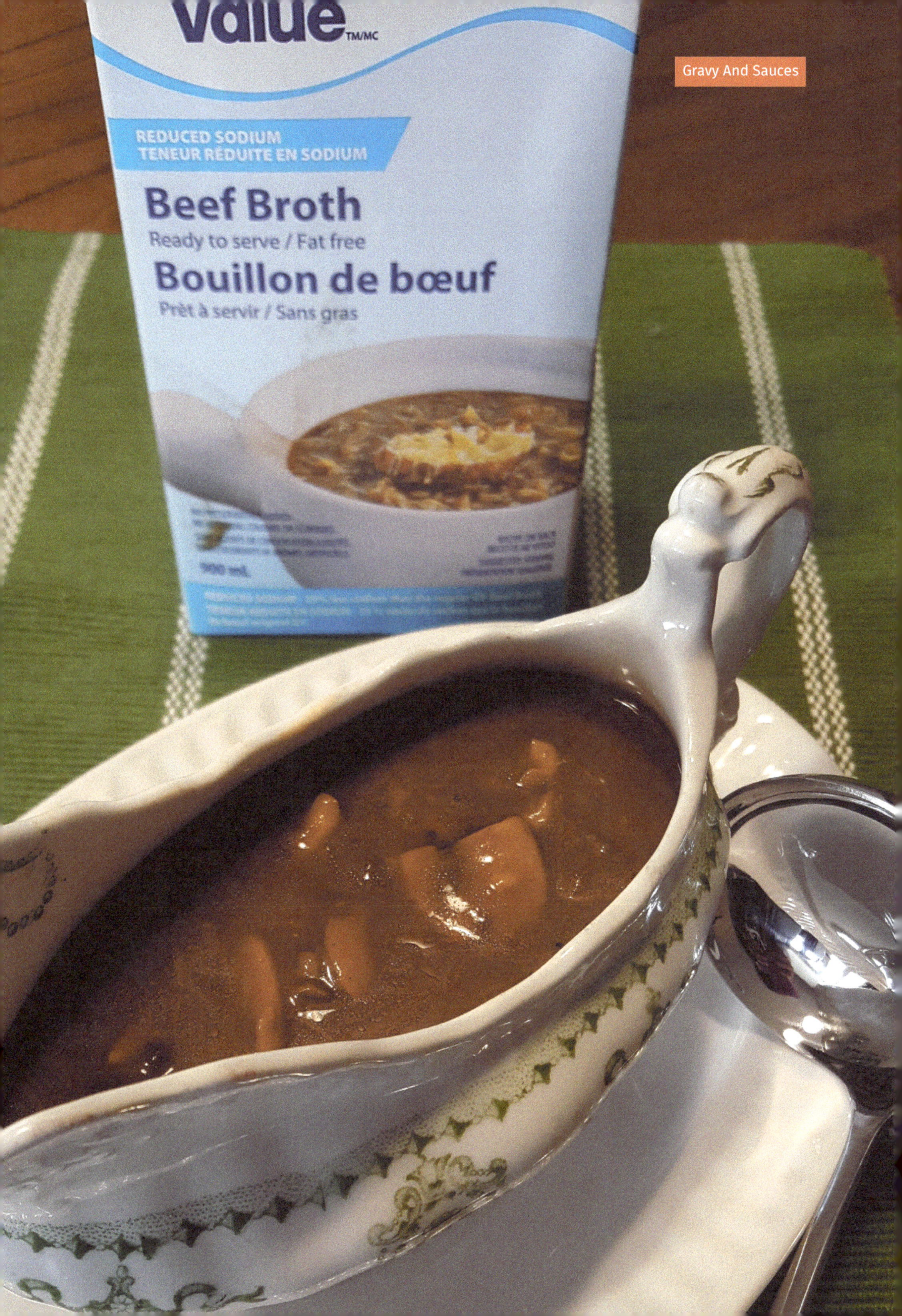

Beef Broth
Ready to serve / Fat free
Bouillon de bœuf
Prêt à servir / Sans gras

REDUCED SODIUM
TENEUR RÉDUITE EN SODIUM

CHICKEN GRAVY

This gravy is liquid gold. It is what makes the Comfort Chicken Bowl (page 100) and other recipes complete and utterly awesome.

INGREDIENTS

1 package chicken or turkey gravy mix (I use Knorr)

¾ c. low-sodium chicken broth

½ c. low-fat milk (I use ¼ c. unsweetened almond milk plus ¼ c. low fat milk)

1 t. butter

½ t. poultry seasoning

½ t. dried thyme

¼ t. or more ground black pepper

INSTRUCTIONS

1. In a small pot, combine broth, milk, spices, and gravy mix. Turn heat to medium–high and whisk until it boils and thickens. Cook for one to two minutes.

2. Remove from heat and add the butter, stirring till it melts.

3. Enjoy your gravy!

NOTE: If you have pan drippings from making a turkey or roasted chicken, use the drippings in place of the chicken broth. Make sure it equals about a three-quarter cup, and, if it doesn't, make up the difference with chicken broth.

Gravy And Sauces

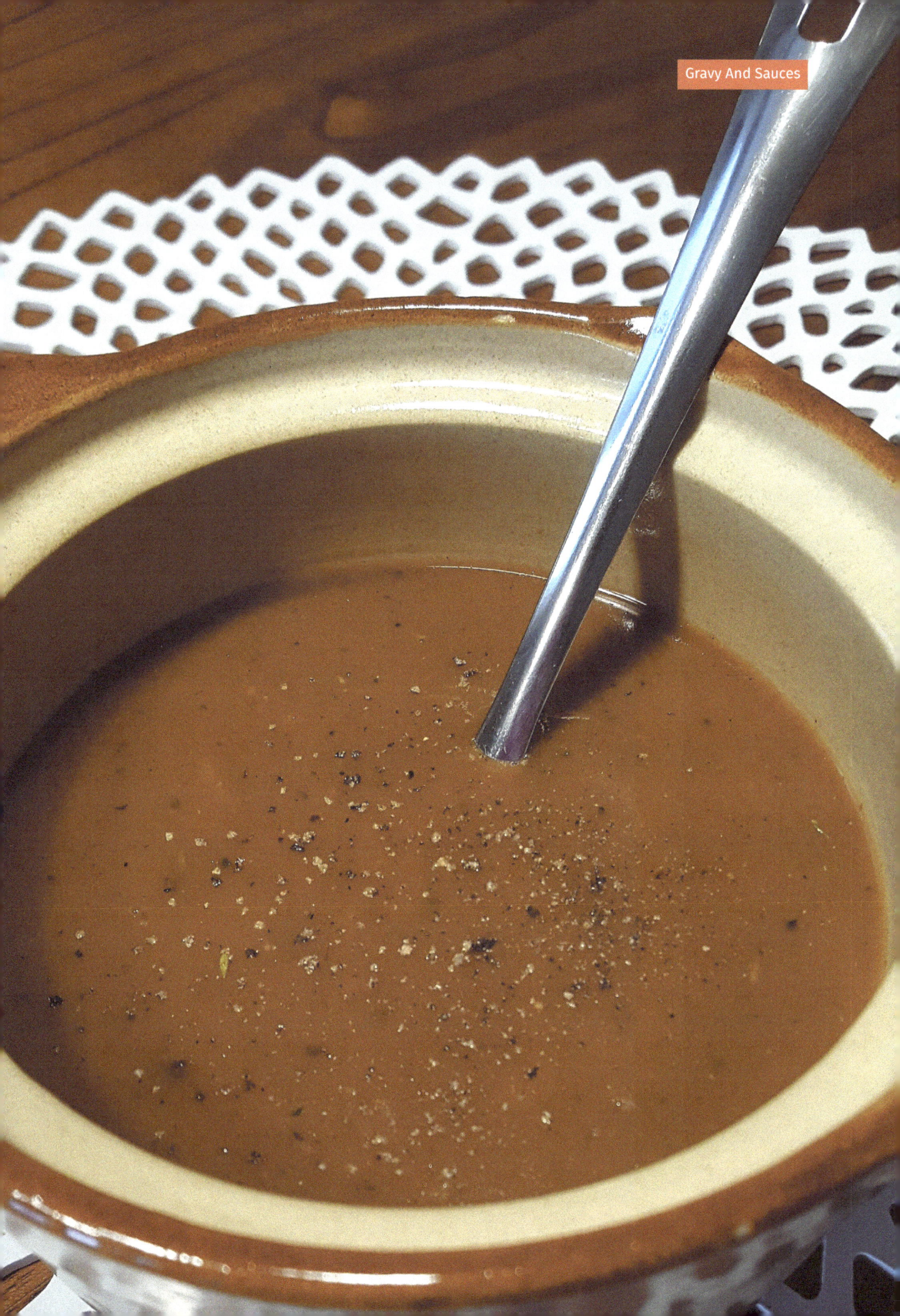

NO-SUGAR BBQ SAUCE

Years ago, I remember trying to make a no-sugar BBQ sauce and it never tasted right. Thanks to no-sugar-added ketchup, it's easier than ever to duplicate the taste of a commercial bottled one. Don't be afraid of the long list of ingredients, as it will be well worth it! You will be making this often, especially during grilling season!

INGREDIENTS

- 2 c. no-sugar-added ketchup (I use Heinz)
- 3 T. chili powder
- 3 T. yellow mustard
- ¾ c. sugar-free apricot preserves (I use no-sugar-added Smucker's)
- 2 T. sugar-free maple syrup
- 2 T. liquid smoke
- 1 t. garlic powder
- 1 t. onion powder
- 1 t. paprika
- ½ t. black pepper
- 2 T. Truvia Brown Sugar Blend
- 1 t. hot sauce (I use Frank's)
- 1 T. Worcestershire sauce

INSTRUCTIONS

1. In a medium-sized pot, simmer all the above ingredients over medium heat for 15 minutes, stirring occasionally.
2. Remove from heat and allow to cool. Store in the refrigerator in a jar or bottle.

NOTE: If you prefer more kick to your BBQ sauce, add one-quarter teaspoon cayenne pepper to the pot.

Gravy And Sauces

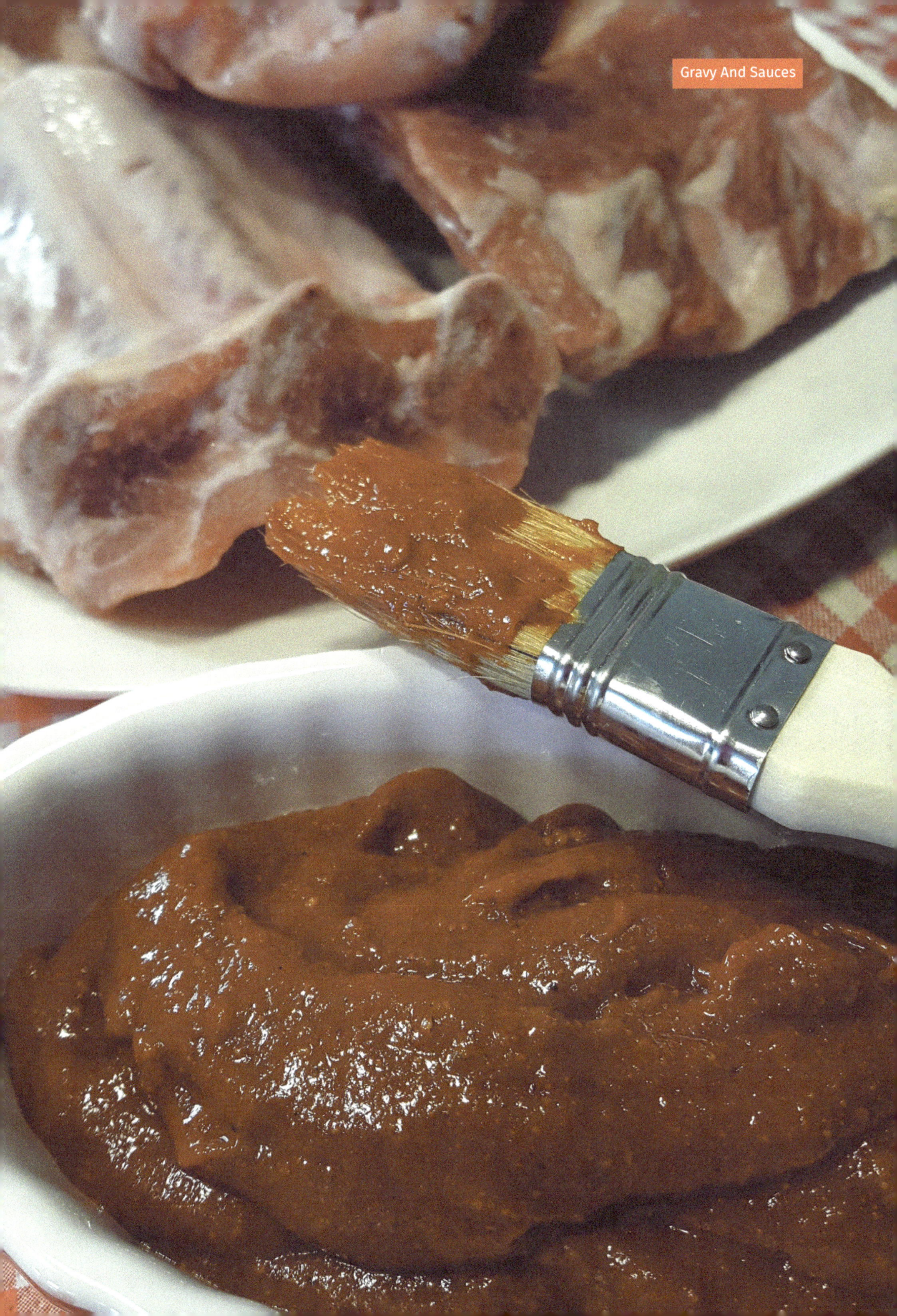

BLUEBERRY SAUCE

This is an outstanding recipe that is so versatile. You can use it as a topping for sugar-free cheesecake or dessert crêpes, or you can put a nice dollop of it on plain Greek yogurt. If you sneak a spoonful right from the fridge, that's just fine, too! Yum.

INGREDIENTS

- 3 c. frozen blueberries (make sure there is no added sugar)
- ¼ c. Truvia Baking Blend
- 2 t. lemon juice
- 1 t. lemon zest
- 2 t. cornstarch (mixed with about 1 t. water to form a smooth white liquid)
- Pinch of salt

INSTRUCTIONS

1. In a medium-sized pot, combine all ingredients, except the cornstarch.
2. Heat on medium–high, stirring occasionally, until berries are thawed and begin to boil. Turn heat down to a low simmer and continue to cook for one minute.
3. Add the cornstarch mixture and stir continuously as it cooks and thickens. Boil for about one minute, then remove from heat.
4. Taste and adjust to your liking. If you like it more tart, you can add some extra lemon juice. If it isn't sweet enough, go ahead and add a bit more Truvia, but do it very gradually as you might not need very much. Start with one-quarter teaspoon at a time.
5. <u>Million-dollar tip</u>: I usually add a squirt or two of a flavoured water enhancer, such as raspberry or blueberry. This is optional, but I find that it adds an amazing depth to the fruit without any added calories or carbs. Cool in the pot and transfer to a mason jar or other closed container and store in the fridge.
6. Make this often, so you always have it on hand!

Note: You can also try using different berries. Just swap out the blueberries for cranberries or strawberries, etc.

Gravy And Sauces

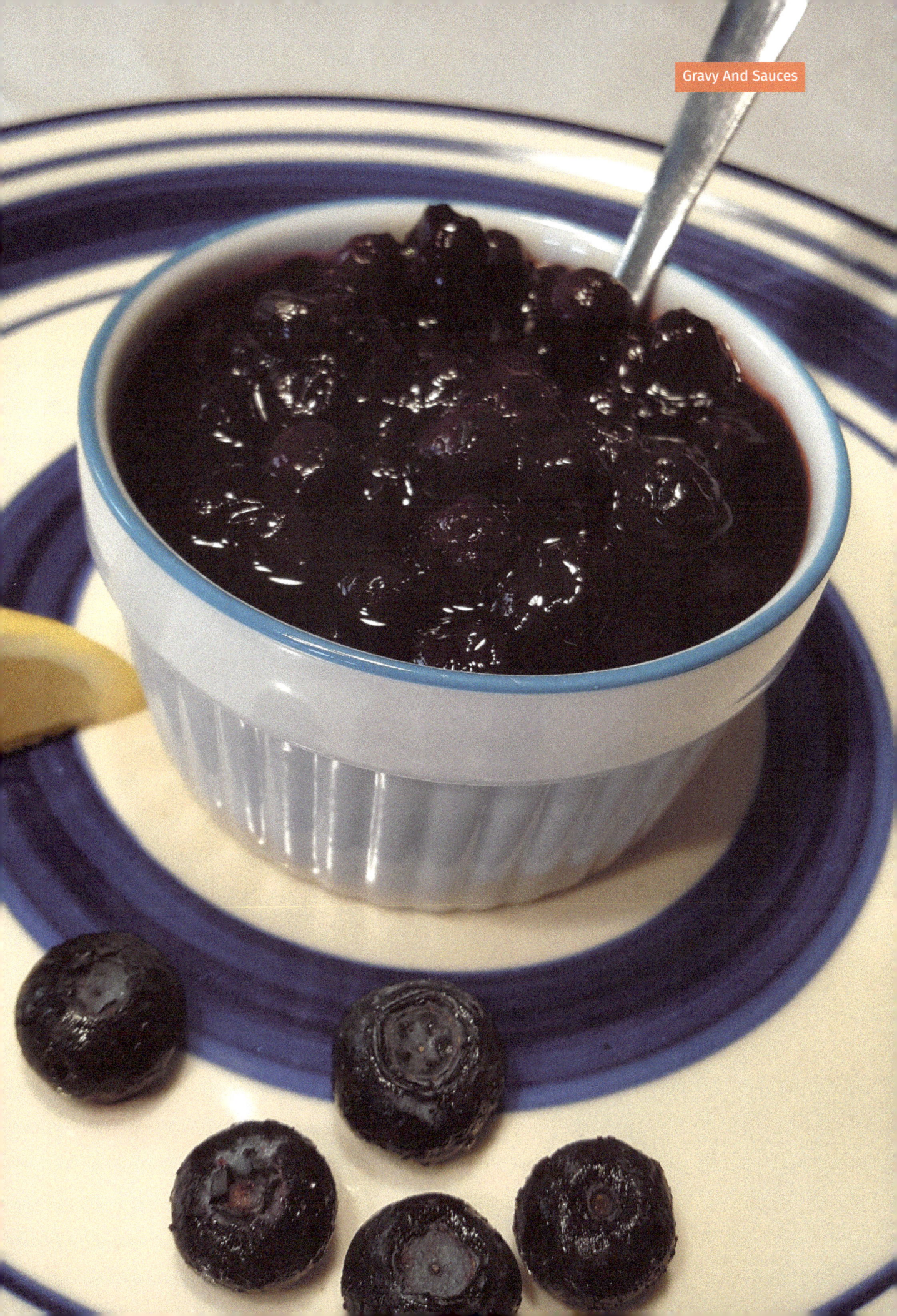

CHOCOLATE DIPPING SAUCE

Who knew that just a few ingredients that we usually have on hand could make such a decadent sauce for dipping luscious strawberries or cubes of cake, fondue style!

INGREDIENTS

- ⅔ c. unsweetened dark cocoa powder
- ¼ t. ground cinnamon
- Pinch of salt
- 1 c. 2% milk
- ½ c. Truvia Baking Blend or 1 c. Stevia granular
- 1 t. vanilla extract
- 2 T. unsalted butter
- 1 T. orange zest

INSTRUCTIONS

1. In a small pot, combine cocoa powder, cinnamon, salt, and milk. Whisk till well blended.
2. Bring to a boil over medium heat, stirring constantly. Stir in Truvia and reduce heat to low and simmer for five to six minutes, stirring frequently, until thick and glossy.
3. Turn off heat then stir in vanilla, butter, and orange zest. Continue stirring until everything is well blended and butter has melted.
4. Cool before using as a dipping sauce.
5. Store in a lidded container in the fridge. Gently warm to serve.

NOTE: Make this your special-occasion dessert or holiday treat and prepare a lovely tray of fresh fruits and cubes of sugar-free cake (recipe found in Desserts). Of course, you would need to double the recipe!

Gravy And Sauces

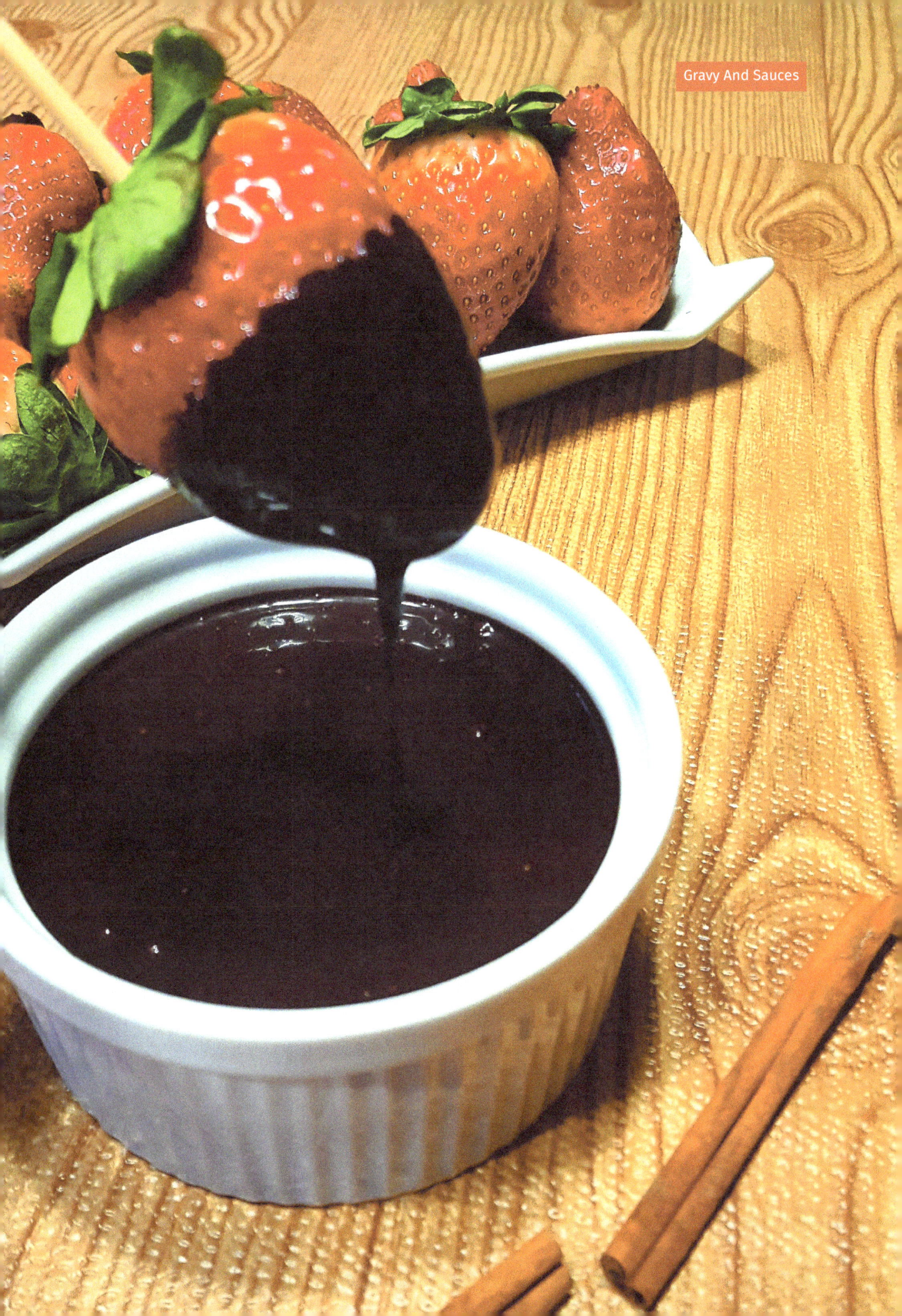

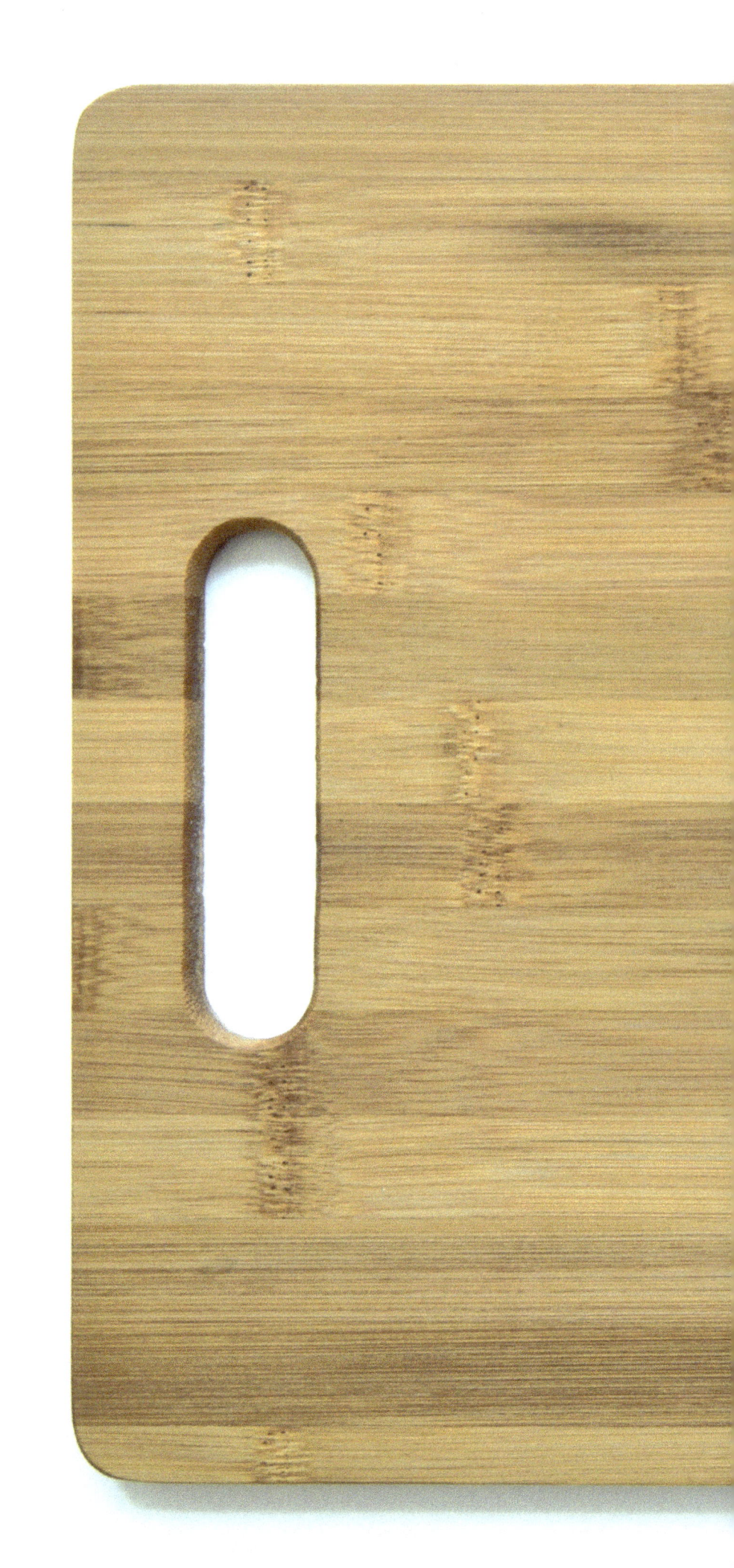

DESSERTS

Pumpkin Pie Mousse 162

Lemon Mousse 164

Chocolate Truffles (No Bake) 166

Chocolate Lover's Decadent Muffins. 168

Oatmeal Poke Cookies. 170

Chocolate Chip Poke Cookies. 172

Biscotti/Mandelbrot 174

Butter Tart Squares 176

Cinnamon Bun Swirl Cake. 178

Lemon Cake With Tart Lemon Frosting. 180

Dessert Crêpes 182

Cheesecake 184

Apple Spice Snack Cake. 186

Old-Fashioned Lemon Meringue Pie. 188

Lemon Lover's Pavlova 190

Best Birthday Cake Ever (All-Occasion Cake). 192

One Awesome Peanut Butter Cookie 194

"Tootsie Roll" Protein Chews 196

Crunchy Protein Cinnamon Cereal. 198

Oh My Strawberry Pie (No Bake) 200

Raspberry Italian Ice 202

PUMPKIN PIE MOUSSE

So simple and so delicious. This is a rich pumpkin mousse without the crust. No need to turn the oven on either. And it's sugar free too!

INGREDIENTS

1 c. whipping cream (unwhipped)

1 1-oz. package of sugar-free butterscotch instant pudding (I use Jell-O brand)

1 c. 1% milk (do not use nut milk as it won't thicken)

1 c. pumpkin puree (not pie filling)

1½ t. pumpkin spice

INSTRUCTIONS

1. Whip the cream until stiff, then set aside.
2. In a separate bowl, beat pudding mix, milk, pumpkin puree, and spices until thick and smooth.
3. Fold in whipped cream. Cover and chill for a few hours.
4. Scoop into dessert dishes and garnish with a dollop of whipped cream or sugar-free Cool Whip. If you want to get fancy and serve this as an elegant dessert, you can pipe the mousse into a martini glass! Don't forget the dollop of whipped cream!

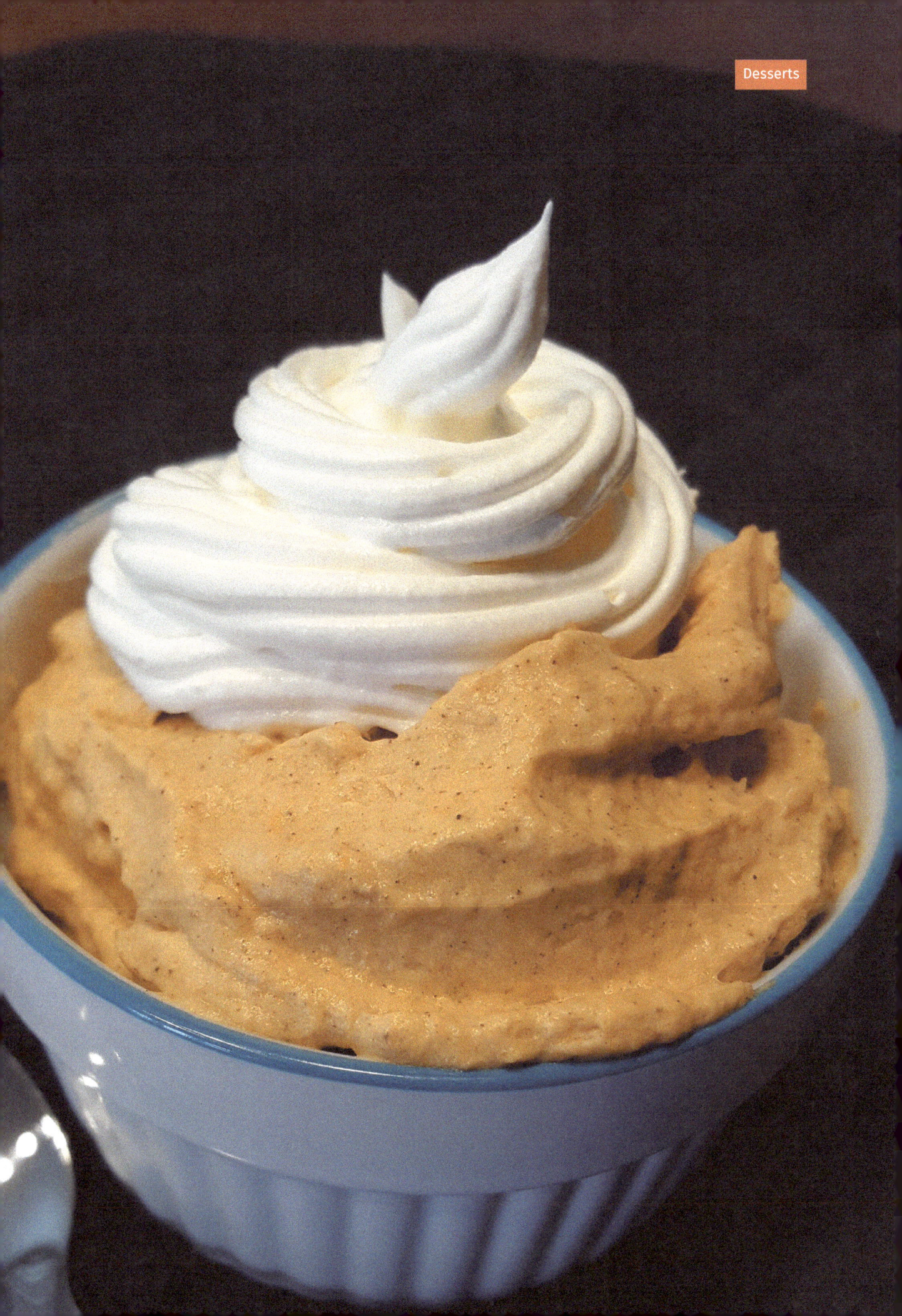

Desserts

COMFORT COOKING
for Bariatric Post-Ops and Everyone Else!

LEMON MOUSSE

Another silly, simple, no-fuss dessert for lemon lovers. You can also use this mousse as a pie filling atop a sugar-free cookie crust.

INGREDIENTS

1 package of sugar-free lemon OR vanilla instant pudding mix

2 c. 1% milk (do not use nut milk)

1 packet sugar-free lemonade powder drink mix, such as Crystal Light (for one pitcher)

½ t. fresh lemon zest

½ tub of sugar-free Cool Whip or about 1 ¼ c. whipping cream, whipped and sweetened to taste with sweetener

INSTRUCTIONS

1. Put pudding mix in a deep bowl, add milk and beat until thick and smooth.
2. Beat in lemonade mix until well combined. Fold in lemon zest, then whipped cream or Cool Whip.
3. Spoon or pipe into lovely glasses and chill well! (Garnish with a dollop of whipped cream.)

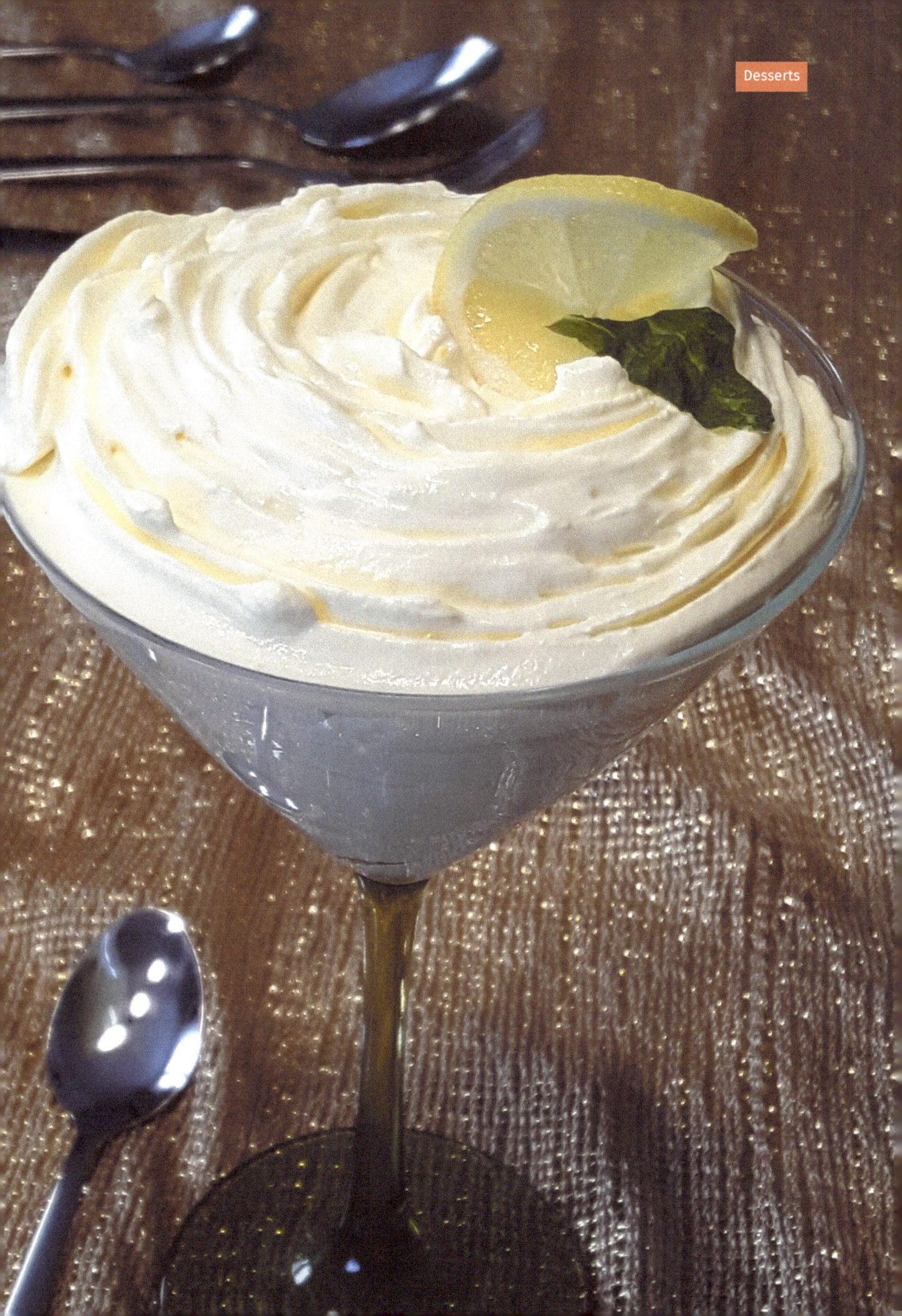

Desserts

COMFORT COOKING
for Bariatric Post-Ops and Everyone Else!

CHOCOLATE TRUFFLES (NO BAKE)

Just a few ingredients and you have velvety-soft, decadent chocolate truffles, perfect for your holiday cookie tray or for gift-giving.

INGREDIENTS

½ c. whipping cream (unwhipped)
6 oz. sugar-free dark chocolate, chopped
3 oz. unsweetened chocolate baking square
1 T. Amaretto, Raspberry, or Orange liqueur
OR Maraschino cherry juice from the jar

Unsweetened cocoa powder, finely chopped walnuts, or unsweetened coconut flakes for rolling

INSTRUCTIONS

1. Heat the unwhipped whipping cream just until it is ready to boil. Remove from heat and add chocolate. Allow to sit undisturbed for two minutes, then stir until smooth.

2. Blend in liqueur or cherry juice. Stir occasionally while it cools to room temperature.

3. Refrigerate until firm, then shape into balls using a small scoop and roll in cocoa powder, nuts, or coconut flakes. Or all three!

TIP: I lightly powder my hands with cocoa powder when rolling to avoid sticking. Make sure you start off with dry hands.

NOTE: To make mocha-tasting truffles, add a few teaspoons of instant coffee granules just before adding the chocolate to the cream.

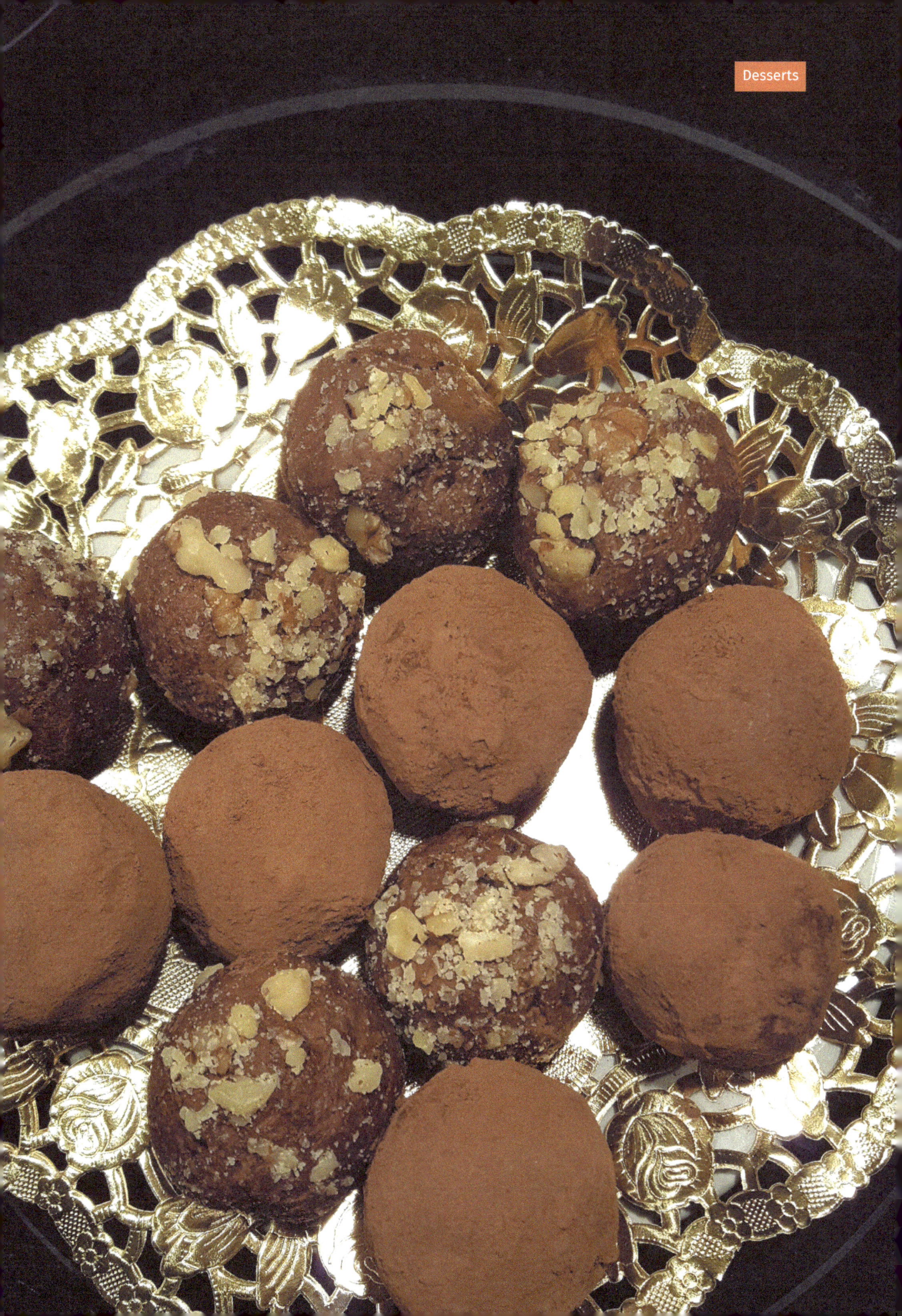

Desserts

COMFORT COOKING
for Bariatric Post-Ops and Everyone Else!

CHOCOLATE LOVER'S DECADENT MUFFINS

When you need a good chocolate fix, this is it. I like the built-in portion control of a muffin, and you will find that one of these muffins is just right! These eggless muffins are moist and chocolatey. They will not disappoint.

INGREDIENTS

Makes 10 muffins

- 1 c. flour
- ½ c. almond flour
- ⅓ c. unsweetened dark cocoa powder
- 1 t. baking soda
- ½ c. plus 2 T. Truvia Baking Blend
- ¼ t. salt
- 5 T. butter, melted
- 1 c. cold coffee (3 t. instant coffee granules)
- 1½ t. vanilla extract
- 1 T. white vinegar
- 2 T. sugar-free, semi-sweet chocolate chips, slightly chopped

INSTRUCTIONS

Pre-heat oven to 350°F.

1. Spray muffin tin with cooking spray. Using two separate bowls, mix dry ingredients into one and wet ingredients into the other. Add the wet ingredients to the dry in three additions, mixing well after each addition.

2. Spoon mixture about halfway up muffin tin (about two tablespoons per muffin).

3. Bake 15 to 20 minutes, until centre comes out clean. Do not overbake.

4. Cool in tin for 10 minutes, then remove onto wire rack and cool completely. Store in the freezer in freezer bags.

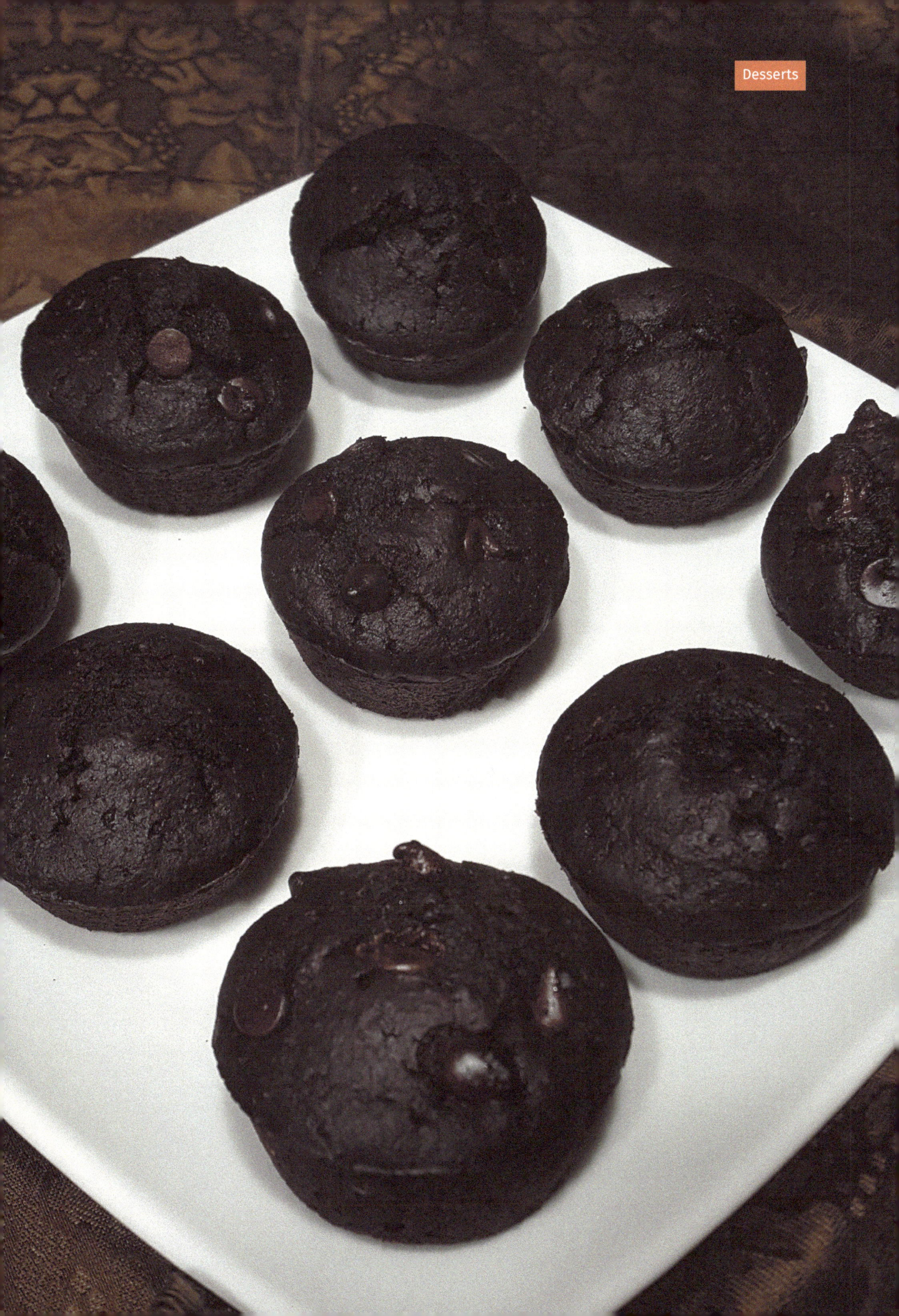

Desserts

OATMEAL POKE COOKIES

I have always loved oatmeal cookies since childhood and Mom perfected her famous "Klara Nugent" cookie, a name we gave to the crispy, flat version that bears our mother's first name. The name "Nugent" was a play on the word nugget, which we amusingly changed to Nugent because we listened to Ted Nugent's music back then. This cookie is a healthier, Truvia-sweetened kind that I know you will love.

INGREDIENTS

- ½ c. white flour
- ¼ c. almond flour
- 1½ c. oats
- ½ t. baking soda
- ½ t. ground cinnamon
- ½ c. soft margarine (I use Becel)
- 1 egg
- ½ t. vanilla extract
- ½ c. Truvia Brown Sugar Blend
- ¼ c. golden raisins, chopped (optional)

INSTRUCTIONS

Pre-heat oven to 375°F and line two cookie sheets with parchment paper.

1. Place dry ingredients, including the raisins, in a small bowl. Whisk to combine then set aside.
2. In another bowl, add margarine, egg, vanilla, and Truvia. Blend well.
3. Add dry ingredients to the wet ingredients and blend until well combined. Drop by heaping teaspoons onto cookie sheet. Bake for eight minutes, then take cookies out and, with a clean finger, poke in three places on each cookie (see NOTE), then return to the oven and bake for an additional three minutes. Cookies should appear slightly under-baked but will firm up as they cool.
4. Cool slightly, then transfer to wire racks. As the cookies air-dry, they will firm up. Place them in an opened cookie jar to harden up, day to day, or close the lid to keep them chewy and moist.

NOTE: I discovered that poking the cookie disrupts the leavening agent, which results in a cookie that has denser areas within the same cookie, almost like a brownie texture. I first saw this when I was back in junior high school and my best friend did this to her cookies every time. I don't think she knew the science behind it but her cookies were always the best.

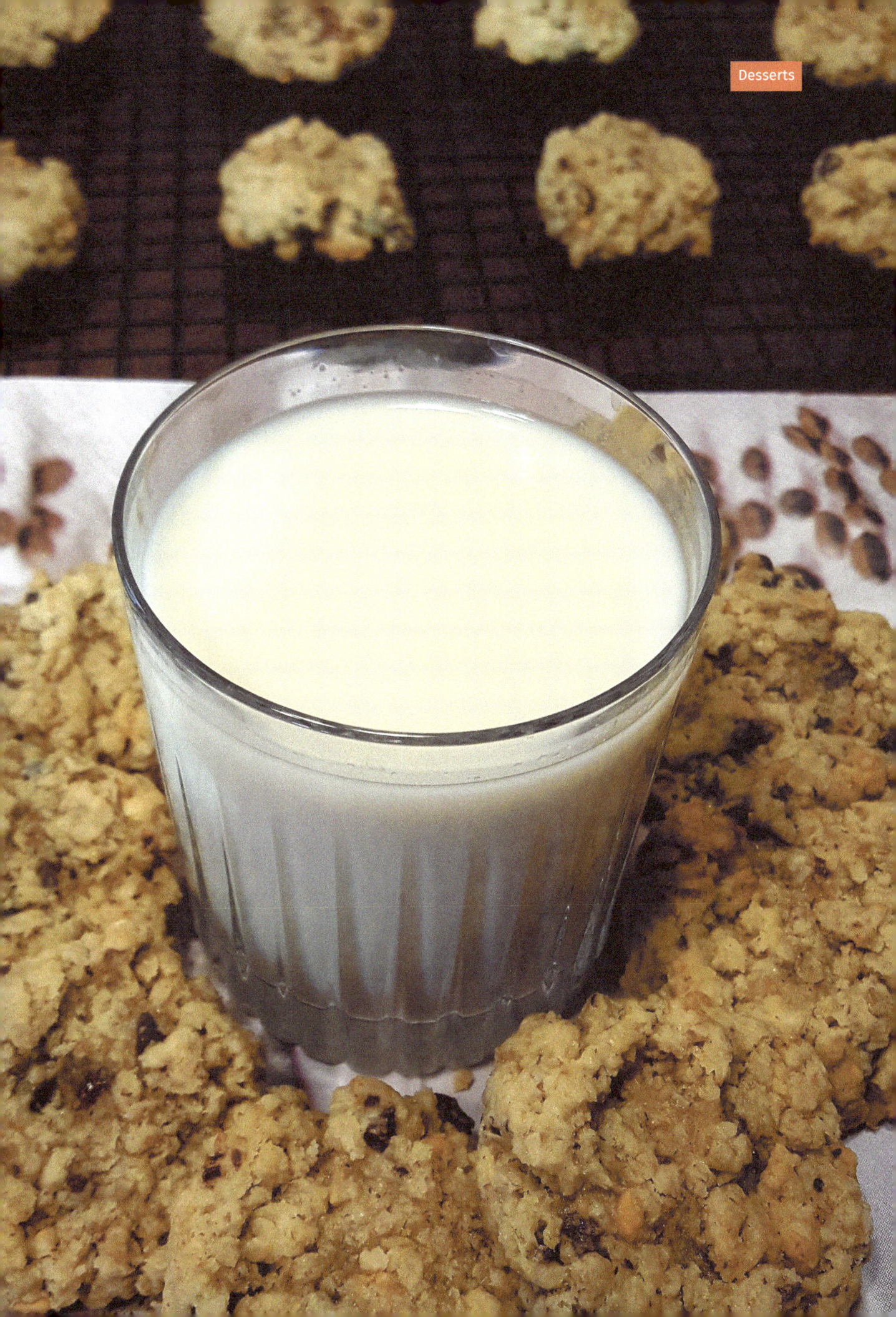

Desserts

CHOCOLATE CHIP POKE COOKIES

I would bet that this is better than any chocolate chip recipe you have been making. Try it soon, and tell me if I am right.

INGREDIENTS

⅔ c. white flour

⅔ c. almond flour

½ t. baking soda

¼ t. salt

½ c. soft margarine (I use Becel)

½ c. Truvia Brown Sugar Blend OR ¼ c. Truvia Brown plus ¼ c. Truvia Baking Blend

1 egg

½ t. vanilla extract

½ c. sugar-free chocolate chips, chopped slightly

INSTRUCTIONS

Pre-heat oven to 375°F and line two cookie sheets with parchment paper.

1. Place dry ingredients in a small bowl. Whisk to combine then set aside.

2. In another bowl, combine margarine, Truvia, egg, and vanilla. Blend well.

3. Add dry ingredients to the wet ingredients and blend until well combined. Fold in chocolate chips, making sure they are well distributed.

4. Drop by heaping teaspoons onto cookie sheet. Bake for eight minutes, then take cookies out and, with a clean finger, poke in three places on each cookie (see NOTE), then return to the oven and bake for an additional three minutes. Cookies should appear slightly under-baked but will firm up as they cool.

5. Cool slightly, then transfer to wire racks. As the cookies air-dry, they will firm up. Place them in an opened cookie jar to harden up, day to day, or close the lid to keep them chewy and moist.

NOTE: Read the science behind finger-poking in notes for Oatmeal Poke Cookies.

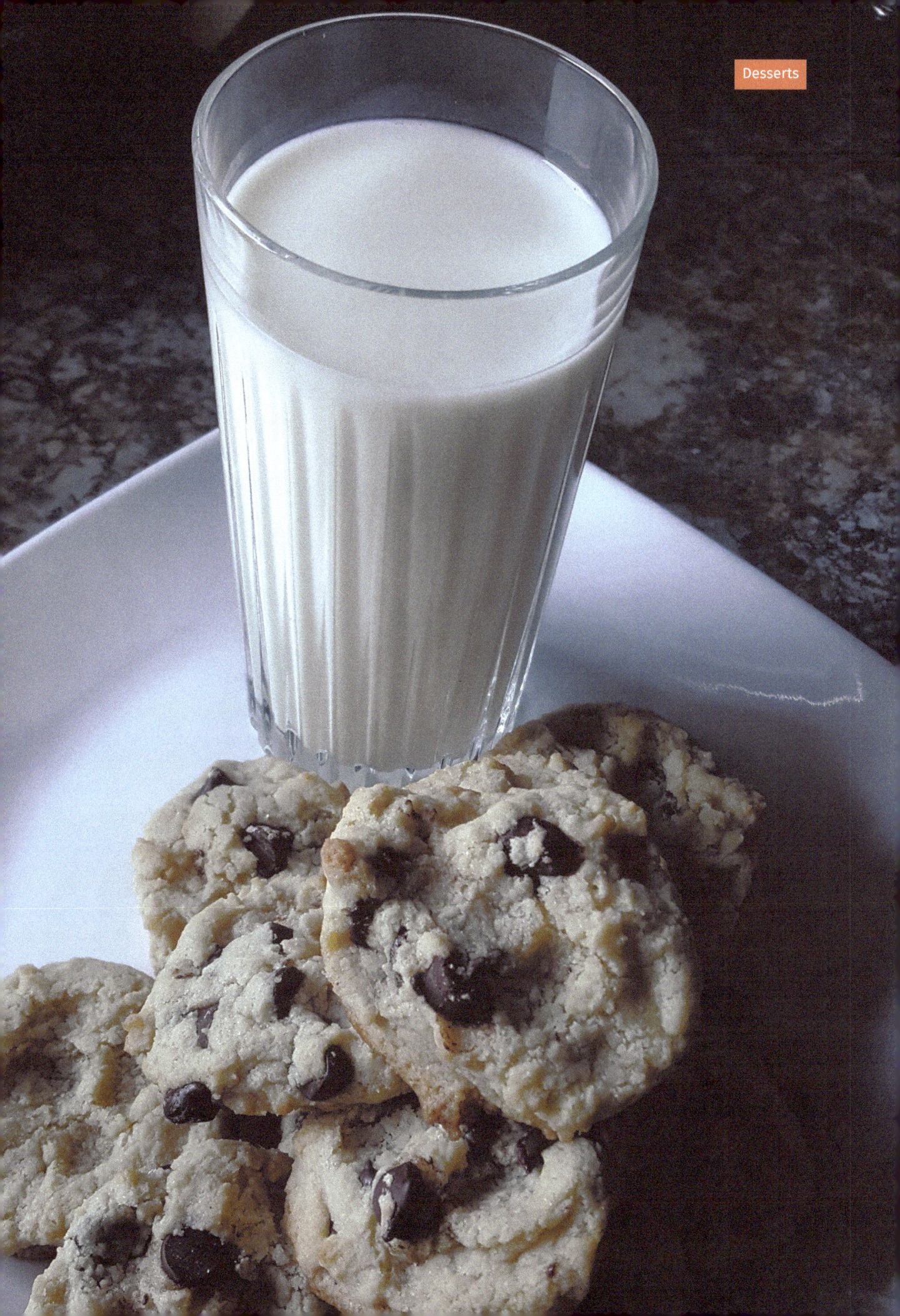

Desserts

BISCOTTI/MANDELBROT

Mandelbrot was the twice-baked cookie that we ate, which is the Jewish version of biscotti. Lately, biscotti has become incredibly fashionable and available in cafes and stores. Make your own! This healthier, no-sugar version is delish and so easy to prepare!

INGREDIENTS

- 1 large egg
- 1 large egg yolk
- ⅔ c. Truvia Baking Blend
- ¼ c. salted butter, melted
- 1 t. vanilla extract
- 1 t. almond extract
- 2 c. almond flour
- ¾ c. white flour
- 1½ t. baking powder
- Pinch of salt
- ¼ c. dried, unsweetened cranberries, chopped (optional)
- ¼ c. pistachios, chopped (optional)
- ¼ c. sugar-free chocolate chips, chopped (optional)

INSTRUCTIONS

Pre-heat oven to 350°F.

1. In a large bowl with a hand mixer, beat together the egg and egg yolk until thick and lemon-coloured. Add Truvia, melted butter, vanilla, and almond extracts and beat on low, until well blended.

2. Mix the two flours, baking powder, and salt together in a small bowl. Add to the egg mixture in three additions, blending well after each addition. Dough will form into a ball.

3. Transfer dough onto a sheet of parchment paper laid out on the counter. Without overworking the dough, knead in the cranberries, pistachios, or chocolate chips, or a combination of two. This is optional; however, it will launch your cookies' flavour beyond the stratosphere!

4. Divide the dough in half, then roll into two logs, measuring about eight inches long by two inches wide. Transfer the logs with the parchment paper onto a cookie sheet. Flatten the logs slightly and, with a knife, score the logs in about quarter-inch-wide slices. You should get roughly 12 cookies per log.

5. Bake for 20 to 25 minutes, until golden brown and firm to the touch. Cool for 15 minutes, then transfer the biscotti to a cutting board and, with a serrated knife, slice each cookie along the score marks. They should be roughly about one-half inch wide after baking.

6. Arrange the slices on the cookie sheet and bake for eight to ten minutes, at 350°F, until browned. Remove from the oven and turn the cookies over and bake an additional three minutes.

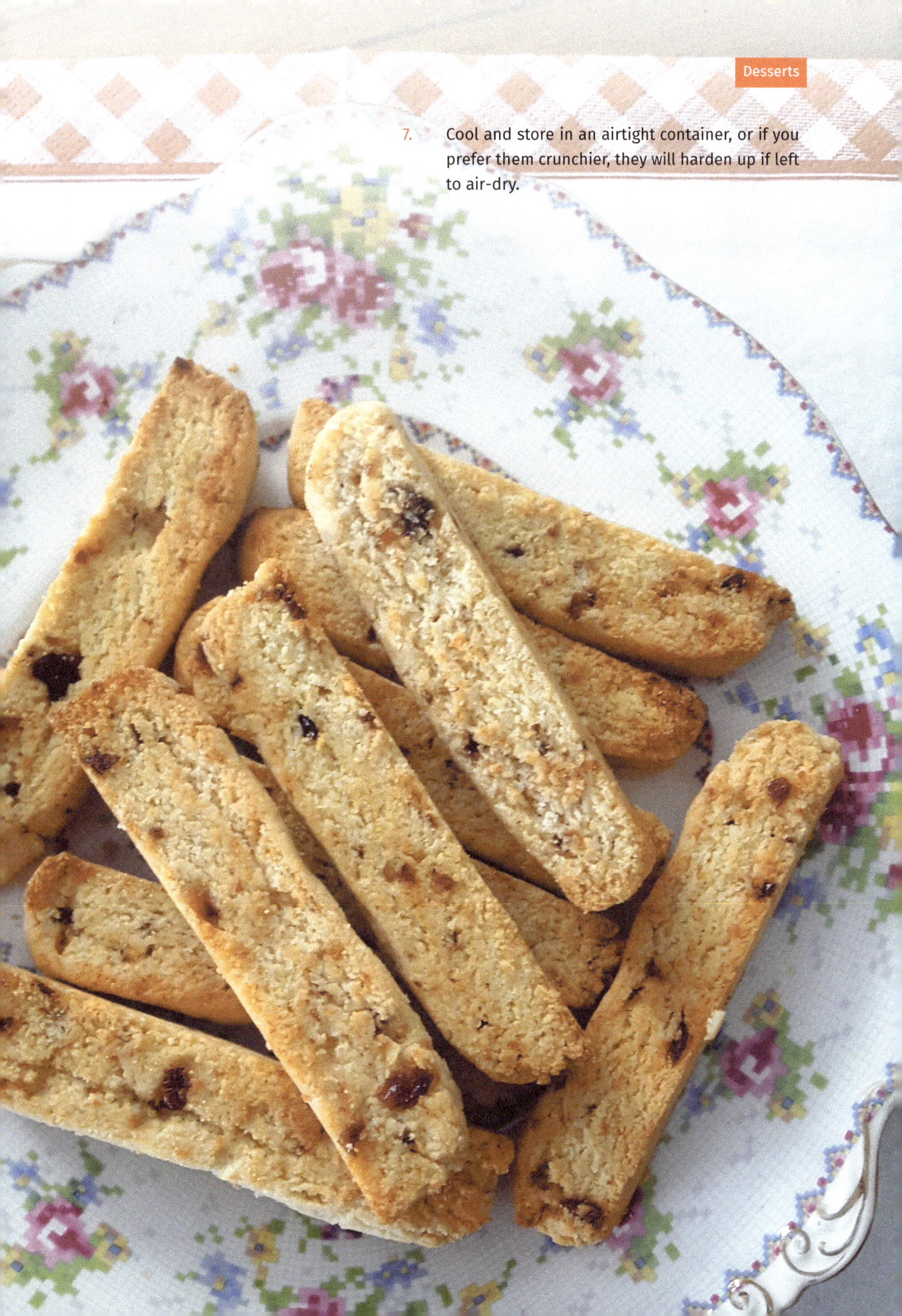

Desserts

7. Cool and store in an airtight container, or if you prefer them crunchier, they will harden up if left to air-dry.

COMFORT COOKING
for Bariatric Post-Ops and Everyone Else!

BUTTER TART SQUARES

Ellen, a good friend of mine, is a butter tart "maven." I told her that I was working on a butter tart recipe that would be "Ellen-worthy." When I finally got the recipe just right, I snapped a photo of it and sent it to her. She could not taste it in that moment, but I think the picture was enough to stir the salivary glands as I received a one-word text back, "Awesome." Since then, Ellen has had the chance to bake up this square and can also verify its fabulous taste and texture!

FOR CRUST

½ c. unsalted butter, room temperature
½ c. almond flour
¾ c. white flour

2 T. Truvia Brown Sugar Blend
Pinch of salt

FOR FILLING

3 eggs
½ c. Truvia Brown Sugar Blend
3 T. white flour
¾ t. baking powder

¼ t. salt
¼ c. pecans or walnuts, chopped (optional)
1½ T. raisins, chopped (optional)

INSTRUCTIONS

1. Combine Crust ingredients in a small bowl and mix well until crumbled. Press into an ungreased 8 × 8 pan and bake at 350°F for 20 minutes, until lightly browned. Cool for 10 minutes.

2. Beat eggs and Truvia, until light and thick. Add remaining Filling ingredients and combine well.

3. Spread Filling evenly over cooled Crust and bake for 12 to 13 minutes. Centre should not be firm; it should appear loose and jiggly. This is the KEY to achieving an ooey-gooey texture. Remove from oven and onto a wire rack to cool completely. Refrigerate to stiffen up a bit before cutting into nine squares. These can be individually frozen in vegetable sprayed foil to avoid sticking.

NOTE: This is in no way a treat that should be eaten too frequently! Remember, there is a lot of butter in it, so enjoy it on occasion without guilt! When you feel like a butter tart—this is still a better option than going to the bakery!

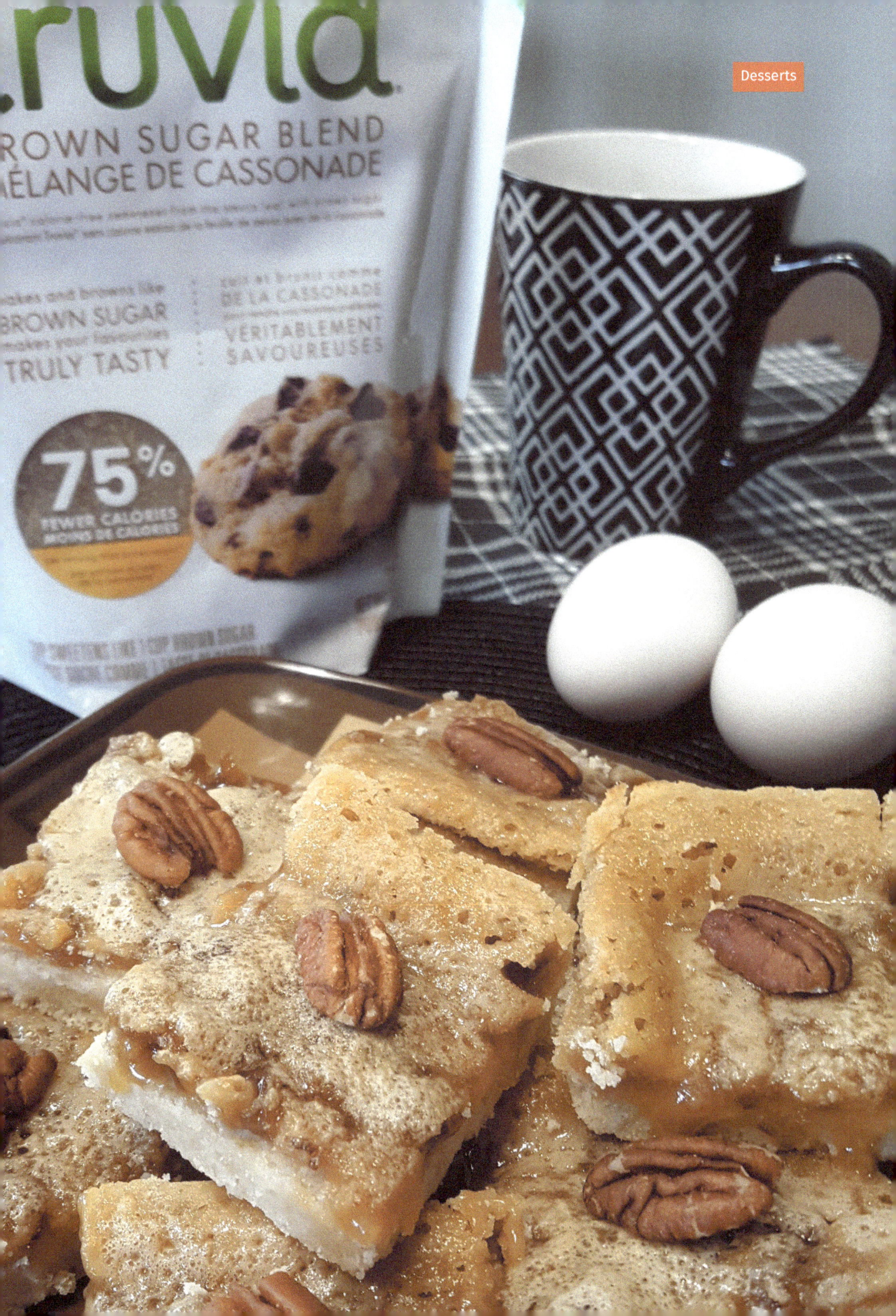

Desserts

COMFORT COOKING
for Bariatric Post-Ops and Everyone Else!

CINNAMON BUN SWIRL CAKE

When you have a craving for a cinnamon bun, this is it! It took me about eight versions of this recipe to finally perfect it. Any hard-core cinnamon bun lover would give it a thumbs-up. Enjoy an occasional piece with a nice cup of coffee. Remember, <u>occasional piece,</u> as it is a butter bomb.

BATTER FOR CAKE

Makes nine squares

A. **Combine in a small-sized bowl and mix well:**

   ¾ c. white flour

   1 c. almond flour

   Pinch of salt

   2 t. plus ½ t. baking powder

B. **Combine in a large-sized bowl and mix until smooth:**

   ½ c. unsalted butter, softened

   ½ c. plus 1 T. Truvia Baking Blend

   1 egg

   1 t. vanilla extract

C. **Combine one-half cup unsweetened almond milk plus one-quarter cup milk with two teaspoons white vinegar in a small bowl. Set aside.**

D. **Cinnamon Topping: Combine one-quarter cup softened salted plus one-quarter cup softened unsalted butter, slightly less than one-half cup Truvia Brown Sugar Blend, one tablespoon white flour, and one heaping tablespoon cinnamon in a small bowl. Set aside.**

E. **Glaze: Combine the following in a small bowl, cover, then allow mixture to slightly stiffen for 15 minutes in the fridge before drizzling squares:**

   1 scoop vanilla protein powder

   1½ T. salted butter, melted

   1½ T. sugar free maple syrup

   ½ t. maple extract

   2 T. Truvia Baking Blend

   1½ T. milk, room temperature

INSTRUCTIONS

Pre-heat oven to 350°F and coat an 8 × 8 glass baking dish with cooking spray.

1. Mix A into B, alternating with C, until well combined. Pour into baking dish and smooth out top evenly. Spoon D on top of cake, spreading evenly from corner to corner. Use a knife to create swirls.

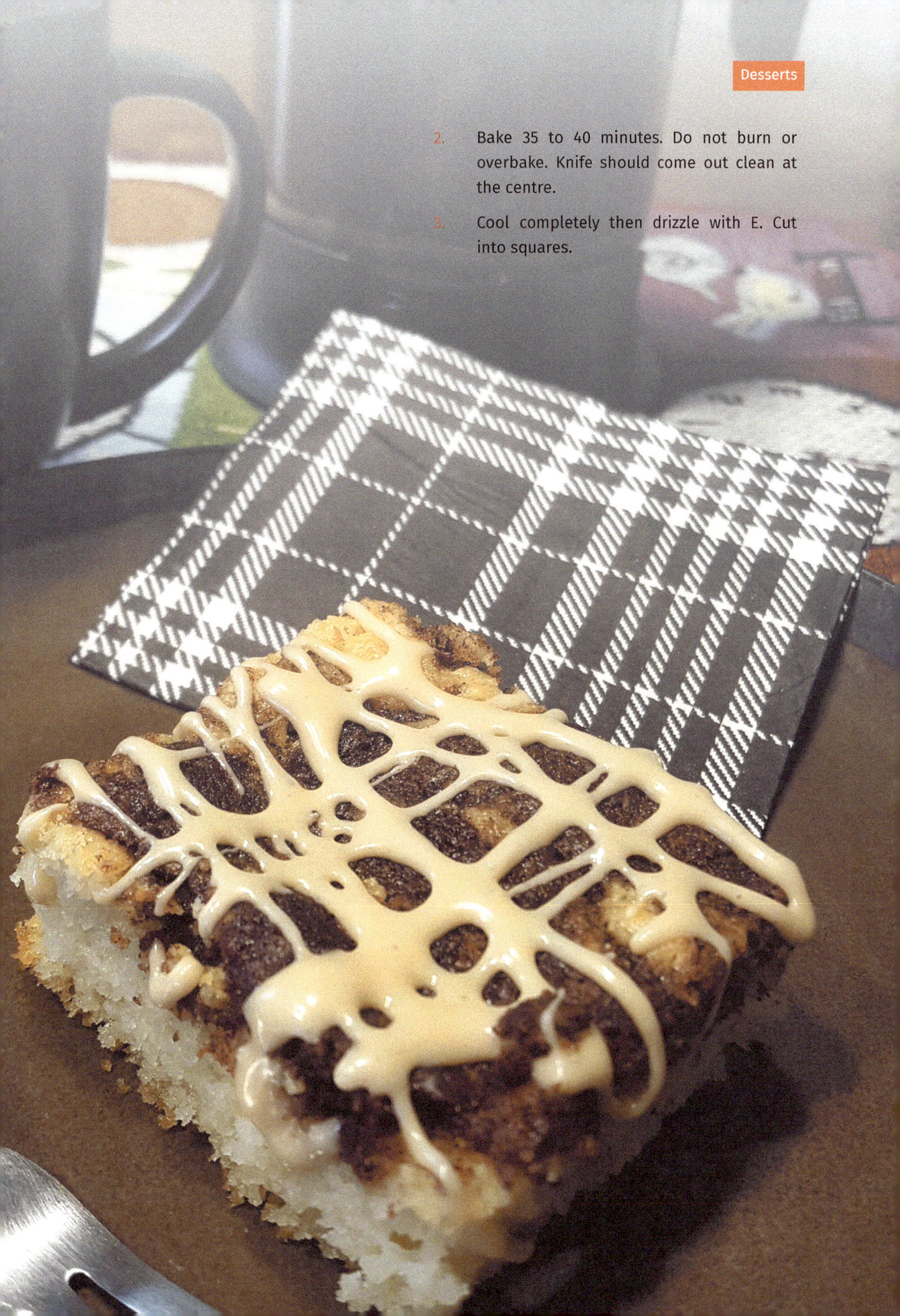

Desserts

2. Bake 35 to 40 minutes. Do not burn or overbake. Knife should come out clean at the centre.

3. Cool completely then drizzle with E. Cut into squares.

COMFORT COOKING
for Bariatric Post-Ops and Everyone Else!

LEMON CAKE WITH TART LEMON FROSTING

Many people love lemony things. This cake is very moist, with a wonderful lemon flavour, and the frosting is lip-smacking tart and even has a little bit of good protein hidden in its creamy goodness.

INGREDIENTS

Makes nine squares

- ½ c. unsalted butter, room temperature
- 3 t. lemon zest
- ½ c. Truvia Baking Blend
- 1 egg, room temperature
- 1 t. lemon extract plus 2 t. lemon juice
- ¾ c. white flour
- 1 c. almond flour
- 2 t. plus a pinch more baking powder
- Pinch of salt
- ½ c. unsweetened almond milk
- ¼ c. milk
- 2 t. white vinegar

FROSTING

- 2 T. unsalted butter, room temperature
- 2 T. no-aroma coconut oil
- 1 t. lemon zest
- 4 T. Truvia Baking Blend
- 4 T. vanilla protein powder
- 2 t. Crystal Light lemonade powder
- 6 t. lemon juice

INSTRUCTIONS

Pre-heat oven to 350°F and spray an 8 × 8 square cake pan with cooking spray.

1. For the Cake, cream butter and Truvia and combine until fluffy. Add egg, extract, zest, and lemon juice, mixing until thoroughly blended.

2. Whisk dry ingredients in a small bowl. Combine almond milk, milk, and vinegar in a small container and let sit for five minutes.

3. Add dry ingredients, alternating with milk mixture, into the egg-butter mixture, stirring well after each addition. Transfer into baking pan, even out the top, and bake for 25 to 30 minutes, or until knife comes out clean from the centre. Do not overbake! Allow to cool completely before frosting.

4. Combine Frosting ingredients and whip until fluffy. Frost your cake thinly. Freeze leftover frosting for another time! Enjoy!

LISA SHARON BELKIN

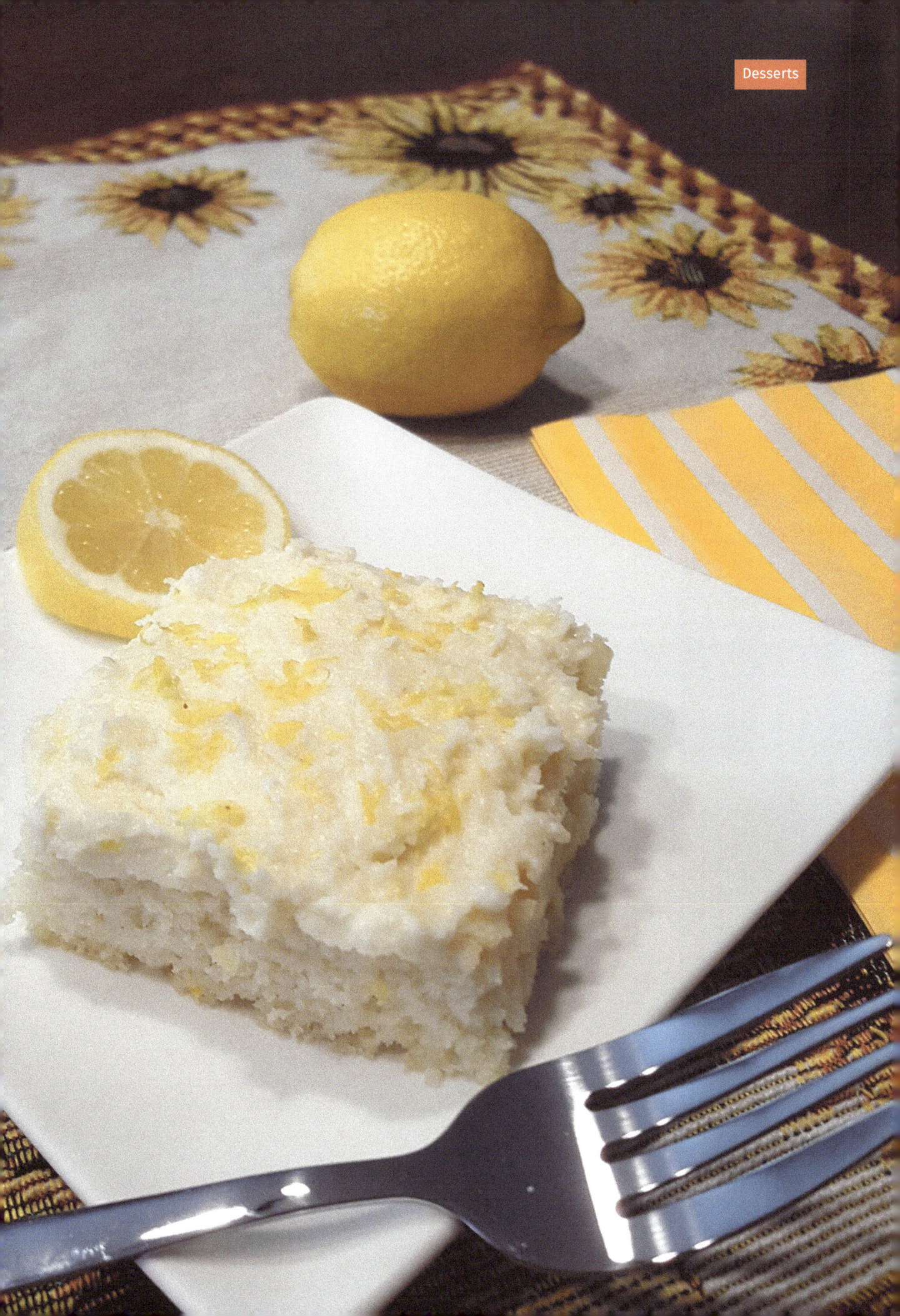

Desserts

DESSERT CRÊPES

These are wonderful as a Sunday brunch menu item or a light dessert. They are versatile, and can be filled with sweetened ricotta cheese, topped with a fruit sauce, or filled with a few teaspoons of fruit sauce, then topped off with a drizzle of no-sugar Chocolate Dipping Sauce. Any way you decide, they are superb!

INGREDIENTS

Makes nine or ten crêpes

- ⅔ c. flour
- ¼ t. salt
- 2 T. granular sweetener (such as Stevia In The Raw)
- 2 eggs
- ¾ c. milk
- 2 T. water
- 1 T. olive oil

INSTRUCTIONS

1. Whisk the wet ingredients together in a medium-sized bowl.
2. Combine the dry ingredients in a small bowl until well combined, then add to the wet ingredients. Cover with plastic wrap and refrigerate for one hour.
3. Heat an 8-inch, non-stick skillet sprayed with cooking spray and proceed to cook crêpes as directed for Low-Carb Crêpes in the "Sides" section.

FILLING SUGGESTIONS

Mix together one cup reduced-fat ricotta cheese (not fat-free), one teaspoon lemon rind, and four tablespoons granular sweetener, such Stevia In The Raw. Fill each crêpe with two teaspoons of filling, then top with any fruit sauce found in Gravy and Sauces, or drizzle with Chocolate Dipping Sauce.

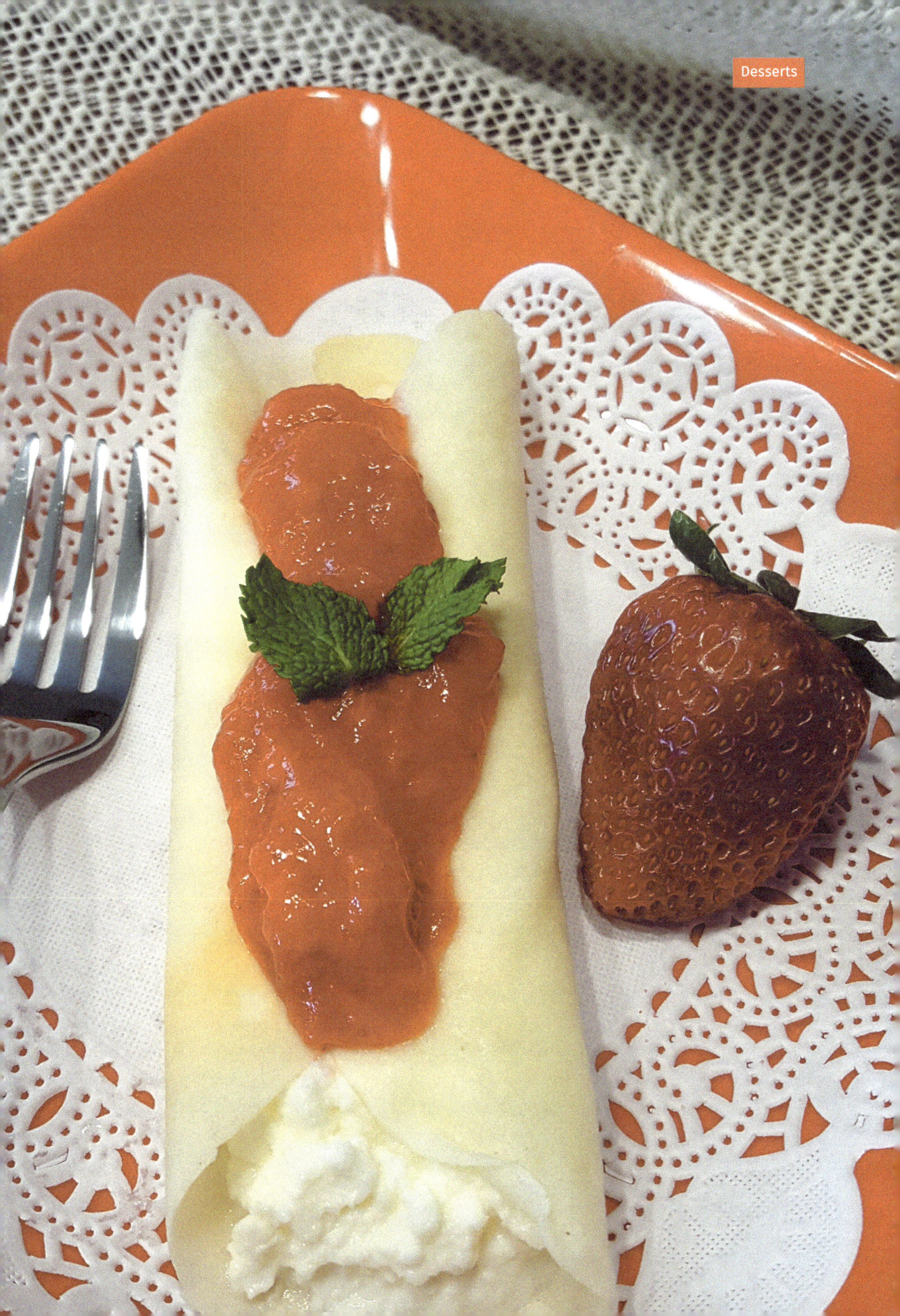

Desserts

CHEESECAKE

Everything that a cheesecake should be. Creamy, dense, and delicious! This is the epitome of dessert after the special-occasion dinner. I often offer to bring dessert to a gathering and I almost always bake a cheesecake. Let this be your contribution to a holiday dessert table!

INGREDIENTS

10 sugar-free oatmeal cookies, crushed and equal to 1¼ c. (I use Voortman's)

4 T. unsalted butter, melted

3 packages reduced-fat cream cheese, room temperature

¼ c. 0% plain Greek Yogurt

¾ c. plus 1 T. Truvia Baking Blend

3 large eggs, room temperature

1 large egg yolk, room temperature

1 t. vanilla extract

1 t. lemon juice

1 T. lemon zest

2 T. white flour

INSTRUCTIONS

Pre-heat oven to 350°F and lightly spray a 9-inch springform pan.

1. Add the melted butter to the crushed cookies and mix well. Press firmly into the bottom of the pan and partly up the sides. Chill crust while preparing the filling.

2. Beat the cream cheese, yogurt, and Truvia at a low speed, until combined. Add eggs one at a time, beating at low speed, to combine. Add egg yolk, flour, extract, lemon juice, and lemon zest, and continue to beat until everything is blended smoothly.

3. Pour the batter on top of the chilled crust. Place on a cookie sheet and bake for 45 to 50 minutes, or until a toothpick inserted in the centre comes out clean. The centre might look a little jiggly—this is okay.

4. Turn off the oven, crack the door slightly open a few inches and allow to cool for one hour.

5. Remove cake from the oven and set it on a wire rack to cool completely. Place a clean paper towel on the top of the cake itself, then cover in plastic wrap and refrigerate for at least five hours, or preferably overnight.

6. When ready to serve, remove the cake from the springform pan onto a lovely cake plate. Cut in small slices and serve topped with Blueberry Sauce (page 156).

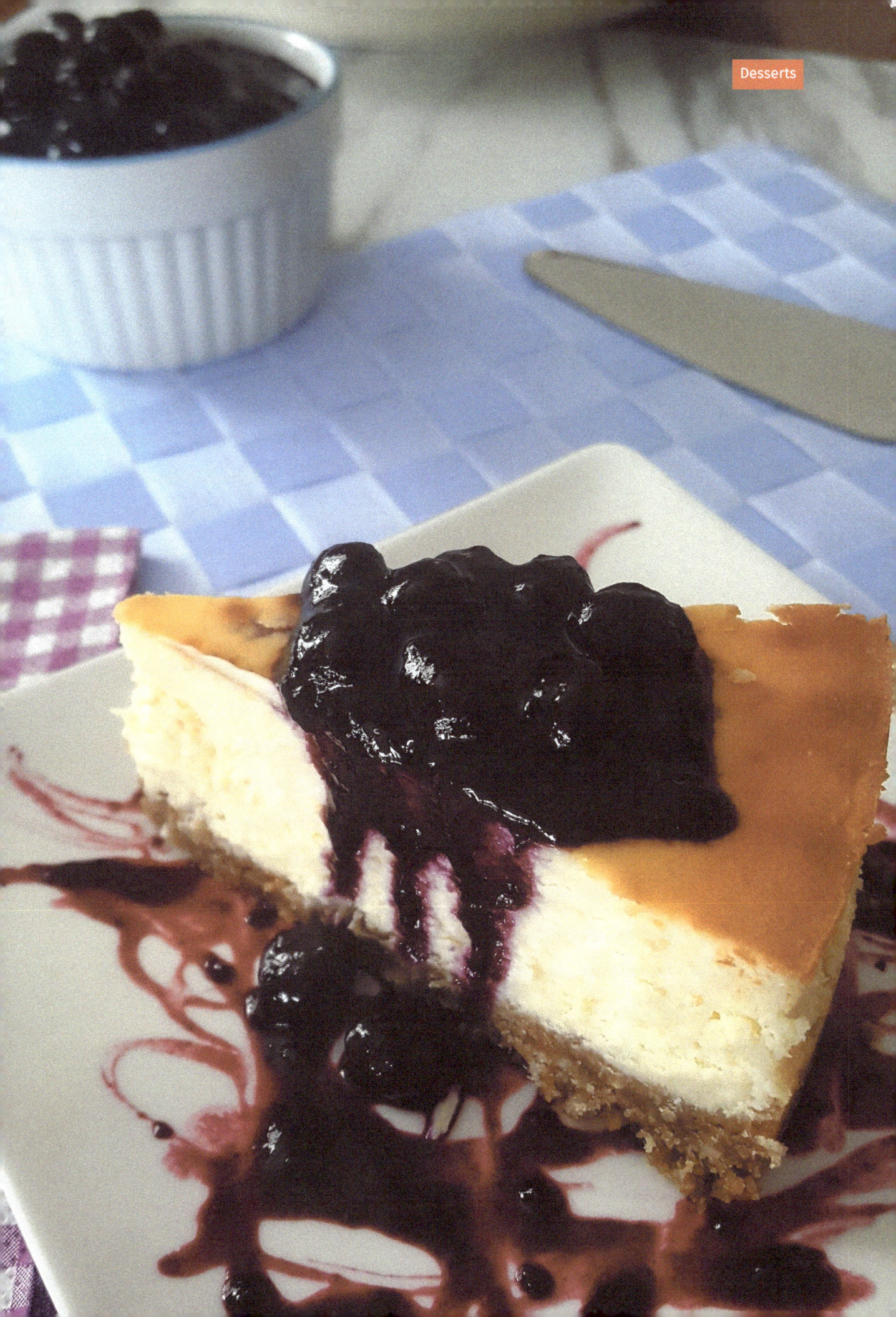

Desserts

APPLE SPICE SNACK CAKE

This is a quick-to-prepare cake that the entire family can enjoy. Bake this up in a snap for unplanned guests, too!

INGREDIENTS

¾ c. white flour

¾ c. almond flour

1 t. baking soda

¼ t. salt

1 t. cinnamon

2 large eggs

½ c. plain 0% Greek yogurt

⅔ c. Truvia Baking Blend

2 medium Granny Smith apples, peeled, cored, and chopped (use a squirt of lemon-ade water enhancer on the chopped apples)

INSTRUCTIONS

Pre-heat oven to 350°F and spray an 8 × 8 square baking dish with cooking spray.

1. Blend all dry ingredients in a large bowl.
2. In a separate smaller bowl, blend eggs, yogurt, and Truvia. Pour wet ingredients into the dry ingredients and stir to combine well.
3. Fold the chopped apples into the batter and pour into baking dish. Even out the top and bake for 25 to 30 minutes, or until centre comes out clean. Cool and cut into squares!

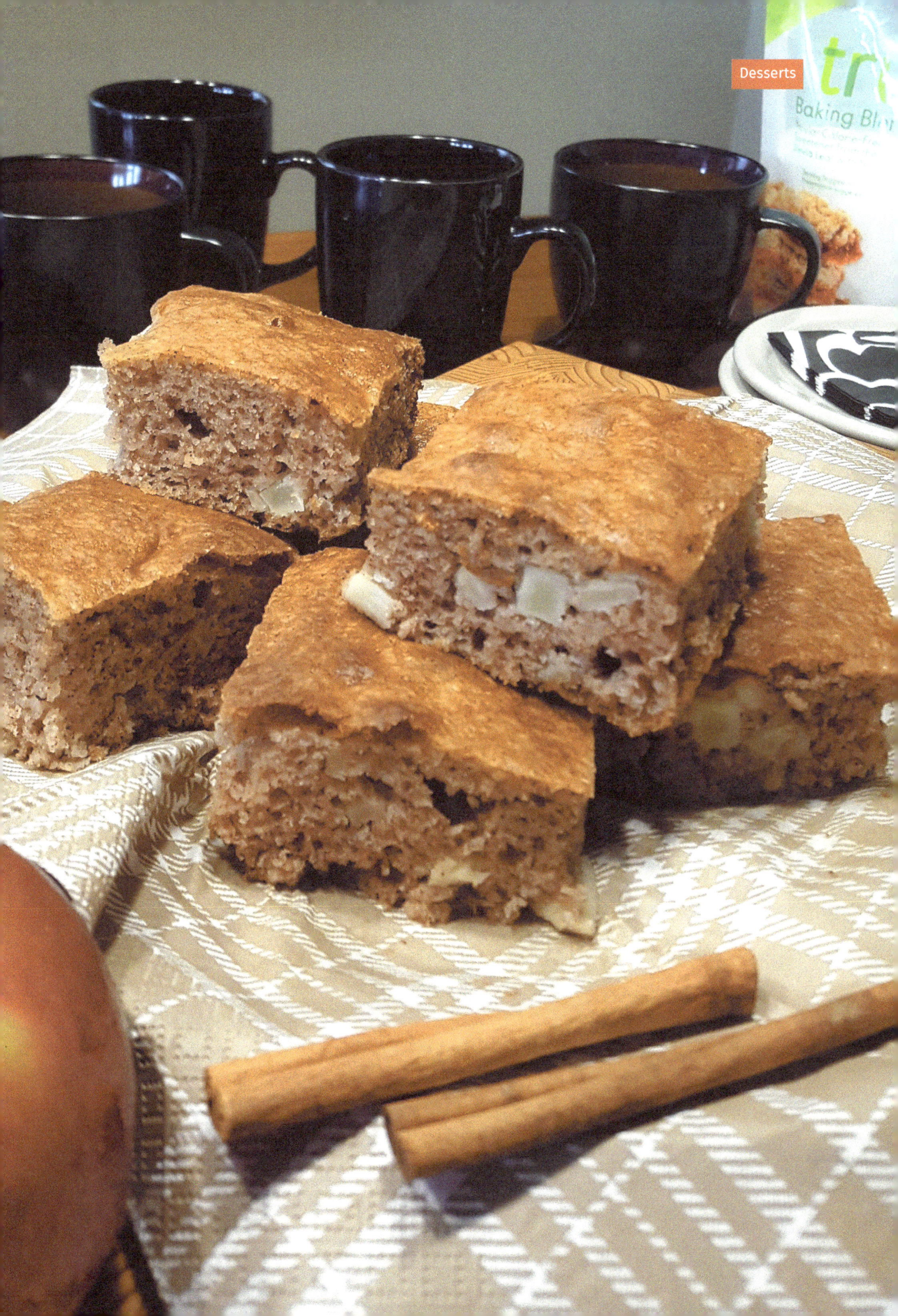

Desserts

COMFORT COOKING
for Bariatric Post-Ops and Everyone Else!

OLD-FASHIONED LEMON MERINGUE PIE

While growing up, we were fortunate to have a family cottage on Lake Winnipeg. In the area was a restaurant famous for their pies. It was here that I was introduced to a lemony dream, which was their traditional lemon meringue pie. I never forgot this place or that pie. Here is my delicious variation on the same theme. Enjoy!

INGREDIENTS FOR FILLING

- 6 egg yolks
- ¼ t. salt
- 1¾ c. water
- 6 T. cornstarch
- ½ c. Truvia Baking Blend
- ½ c. plus 1 T. Stevia In The Raw granular sweetener
- ¾ c. fresh lemon juice
- 1 T. Crystal Light lemonade powder
- 1 T. lemon zest
- 1 ready-made pie shell, baked OR cookie crust (see Oh My Strawberry Pie recipe)

INGREDIENTS FOR MERINGUE

- 5 egg whites, room temperature
- ¼ t. cream of tartar
- 3 T. Stevia granular
- 1 t. vanilla extract

INSTRUCTIONS

1. Place egg yolks and salt in a medium-sized pot and set aside.

2. In a large saucepan, bring water, cornstarch, Truvia, and Stevia to a boil. Stir constantly, as it begins to thicken up after a few minutes. Reduce the heat and add the lemon juice, Crystal Light, and zest, still constantly stirring to combine until it begins to get smooth and glossy. Cook for one minute longer.

3. Remove from heat and slowly start adding the hot mixture into the egg yolks in the other pot, tempering it in small additions while vigorously whisking after each addition so the egg doesn't cook. After the last addition, heat the mixture once again for an additional three minutes, stirring constantly until it thickens.

4. Pour this Filling into a baked and cooled pie shell OR a prepared cookie crust (see Oh My Strawberry Pie crust recipe).

5. Make the meringue. With an electric mixer, whip the egg whites and cream of tartar until soft peaks form. Add Stevia and vanilla. Beat until the mixture becomes thick and glossy. Top the pie, starting at the outer edges toward the middle, dropping by the spoonful.

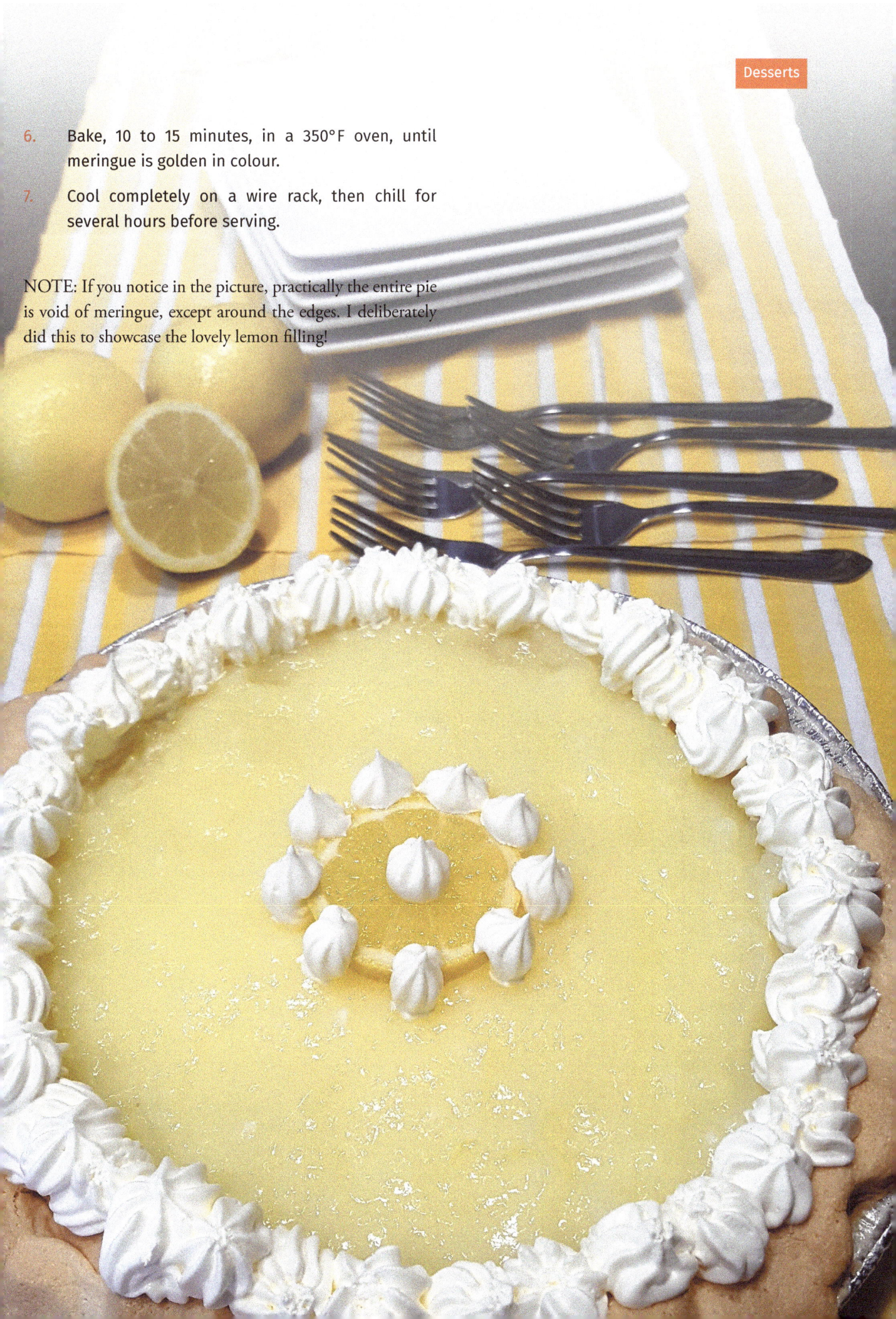

Desserts

6. Bake, 10 to 15 minutes, in a 350°F oven, until meringue is golden in colour.

7. Cool completely on a wire rack, then chill for several hours before serving.

NOTE: If you notice in the picture, practically the entire pie is void of meringue, except around the edges. I deliberately did this to showcase the lovely lemon filling!

LEMON LOVER'S PAVLOVA

This very special dessert, invented in New Zealand, was named after the Russian ballerina Anna Pavlova. The base resembles the bottom of a pillowy white tutu made from meringue, which has a crispy outer edge and a creamy marshmallow centre. Topped with lemony whipped cream and garnished with fruit, it oozes elegance and grace, befitting its name.

INGREDIENTS FOR MERINGUE

- 4 large egg whites, room temperature
- Pinch of salt
- ½ c. Truvia Baking Blend
- 2 t. cornstarch
- 1 t. white vinegar

INGREDIENTS FOR LEMON CREAM

- 2 c. whipping cream
- Packet of whip cream stabilizer (such as Dr. Oetker Whip It)
- 1 T. Truvia Baking Blend
- 4 t. Crystal Light sugar-free lemonade drink mix powder
- 1½ t. lemon zest
- 2 t. lemon juice

INSTRUCTIONS

Pre-heat the oven to 200°F.

1. Place a sheet of parchment paper on a cookie sheet. Using a 9-inch cake pan, trace a 9-inch circle onto the paper. Flip the paper over making sure you can see the traced circle through the paper. Set aside and prepare the Meringue.

2. Beat egg whites with salt in a large bowl with an electric mixer on high speed for about one minute until firm. Slowly add the Truvia and beat until firm peaks form, about two minutes. With a sifter, sprinkle the cornstarch onto the egg whites then add the vinegar. Gently fold everything into the egg whites using a spatula.

3. Spread the meringue onto the parchment circle starting from the middle then moving outward, toward the edges, making a rough disk.

4. Bake for one and a half hours, then turn off the heat and leave the meringue to cool completely in the oven for an additional one hour with the oven door closed. When completely cooled, invert the disk onto a cake plate, peeling away the parchment paper.

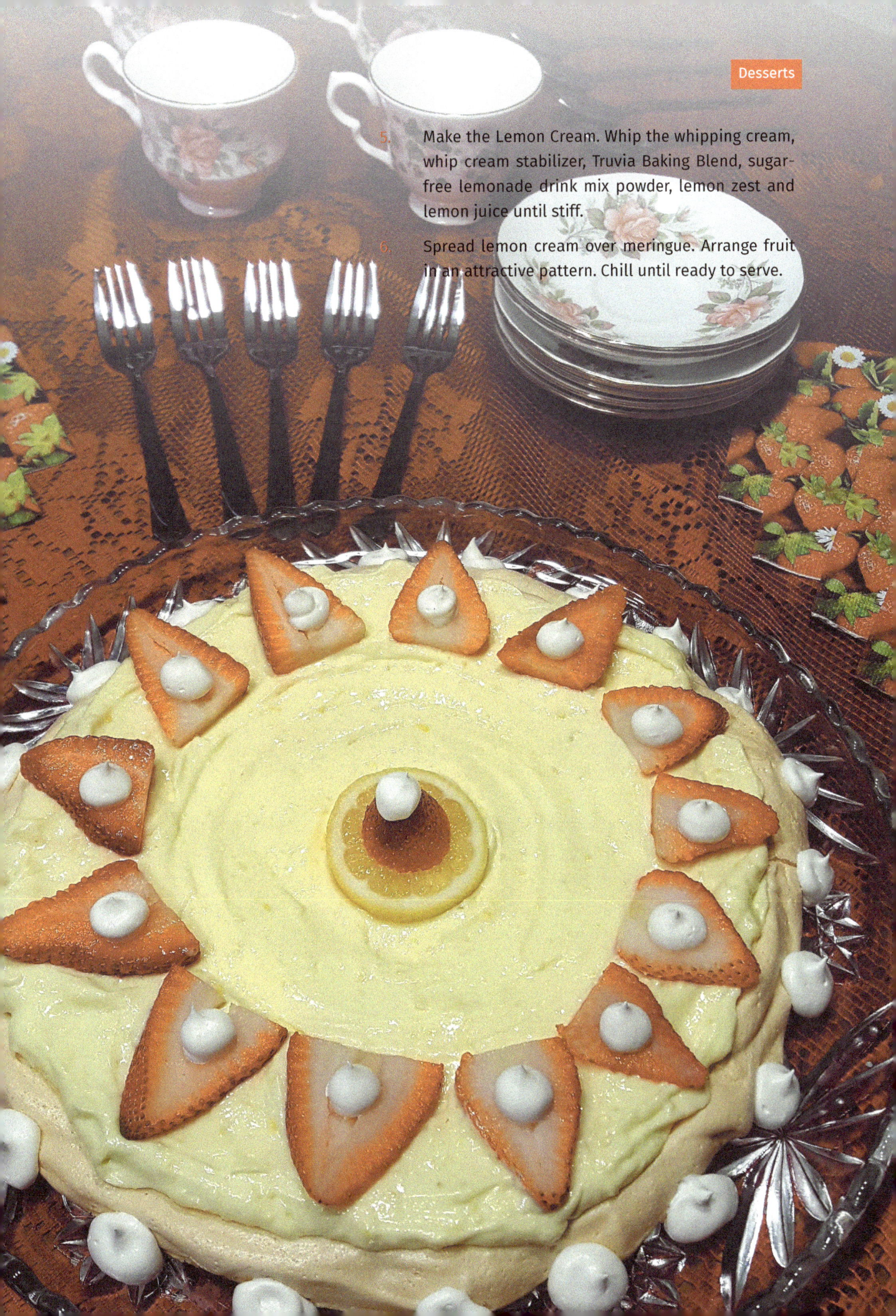

Desserts

5. Make the Lemon Cream. Whip the whipping cream, whip cream stabilizer, Truvia Baking Blend, sugar-free lemonade drink mix powder, lemon zest and lemon juice until stiff.

6. Spread lemon cream over meringue. Arrange fruit in an attractive pattern. Chill until ready to serve.

BEST BIRTHDAY CAKE EVER (ALL-OCCASION CAKE)

Now THIS is a show-stopper of a cake. It is one of the many best surprises in this book. Who would have ever thought that a bariatric-friendly AND delicious birthday cake was even possible?

INGREDIENTS

- 6 eggs, separated
- ½ t. cream of tartar
- ¾ c. Truvia Baking Blend
- ¾ c. almond flour
- ¾ c. white flour
- 1 t. baking powder plus pinch of salt
- 2 t. vanilla extract
- 1 t. lemon juice
- 1 t. lemon zest
- ⅓ c. water
- 2 cups whipping cream (unwhipped)
- 3 T. sugar-free vanilla Jell-O instant pudding mix
- ½ cup no-sugar added apricot preserves (Smucker's)
- 1 t. lemon juice

INSTRUCTIONS

Pre-heat oven to 325°F and spray a 9-inch springform pan lined with parchment.

1. Beat egg whites with cream of tartar until stiff. Set aside. Combine extracts, juice, zest, and water in a small bowl and set aside.

2. Wash off beaters and beat egg yolks till thick and lemon-coloured. Add the sugar, gradually, and blend well. Add the sifted dry ingredients to the egg yolk mixture, alternating with the flavourings and water mixture, beating until well combined.

3. Fold egg whites into the batter, then pour into the springform pan. Bake for 55 to 60 minutes, until lightly browned and knife comes out clean in the centre.

4. Cool for 10 minutes in pan then open latch and allow it to cool on wire rack for one hour. Flip and remove parchment paper and cool completely. Cut cake in half horizontally.

5. Whip two cups of whipping cream with three tablespoons sugar-free Jell-O Vanilla instant pudding mix until thickened.

6. In a small bowl combine one-half cup of no-sugar-added apricot preserves with one teaspoon lemon juice.

Desserts

TO ASSEMBLE

Place half of the cake on a cake stand and spread on the apricot filling evenly. Place top half over bottom half. Add the frosting to the top of the cake by the spoonful, smoothing out the top and continuing halfway down the sides. Garnish with berries just before serving. Happy Birthday!

Variations: Cake is the same. The frosting changes. Strawberry: add strawberry Crystal Light powder to whipping cream and pudding, then mix in sliced strawberries. For chocolate lovers, use sugar-free chocolate pudding powder in the whipping cream and garnish with chocolate shavings and a dusting of granulated coffee. For lemon lovers, add lemonade Crystal Light to the whipping cream, etc. Endless possibilities!

COMFORT COOKING
for Bariatric Post-Ops and Everyone Else!

ONE AWESOME PEANUT BUTTER COOKIE

When you can no longer ignore the need for a peanut butter cookie, this is it. One fantabulous cookie that will hit the spot and won't derail your efforts. Close your eyes while you eat it—then move on.

INGREDIENTS

1 T. regular peanut butter (I use Kraft smooth)

2 T. peanut butter powder

Heaping ½ T. Truvia Brown Sugar Blend

1½ t. egg (mix the egg and measure—refrigerate the rest for another recipe)

INSTRUCTIONS

Pre-heat oven to 350°F.

1. Mix all ingredients in a small bowl. Blend well. Roll with hands into a ball and turn onto a cookie sheet lined with parchment paper. Flatten with the palm of your hand, then, using a fork, press to form the classic imprints with the tines.

2. Bake for 10 to 12 minutes (do not overbake). Allow to cool for five minutes on cookie sheet, then transfer to cool on a wire rack. The longer you wait, the crunchier the cookie will be!

Make 20 peanut butter cookies (in case you've got a crowd)

¾ c. smooth peanut butter

¼ c. peanut butter powder

1 large egg

¼ c. plus 2 T. Truvia Brown Sugar Blend

INSTRUCTIONS

Pre-heat oven to 350°F.

1. Mix ingredients in a medium-sized bowl. Blend well. Roll into small balls about ½ T. of dough for each, then turn onto a cookie sheet lined with parchment paper. Flatten balls with a fork, pressing the tines in two directions to form the classic imprints.

2. Bake 10 to 12 minutes. Allow to cool for five minutes on cookie sheet, then transfer to cool on a wire rack.

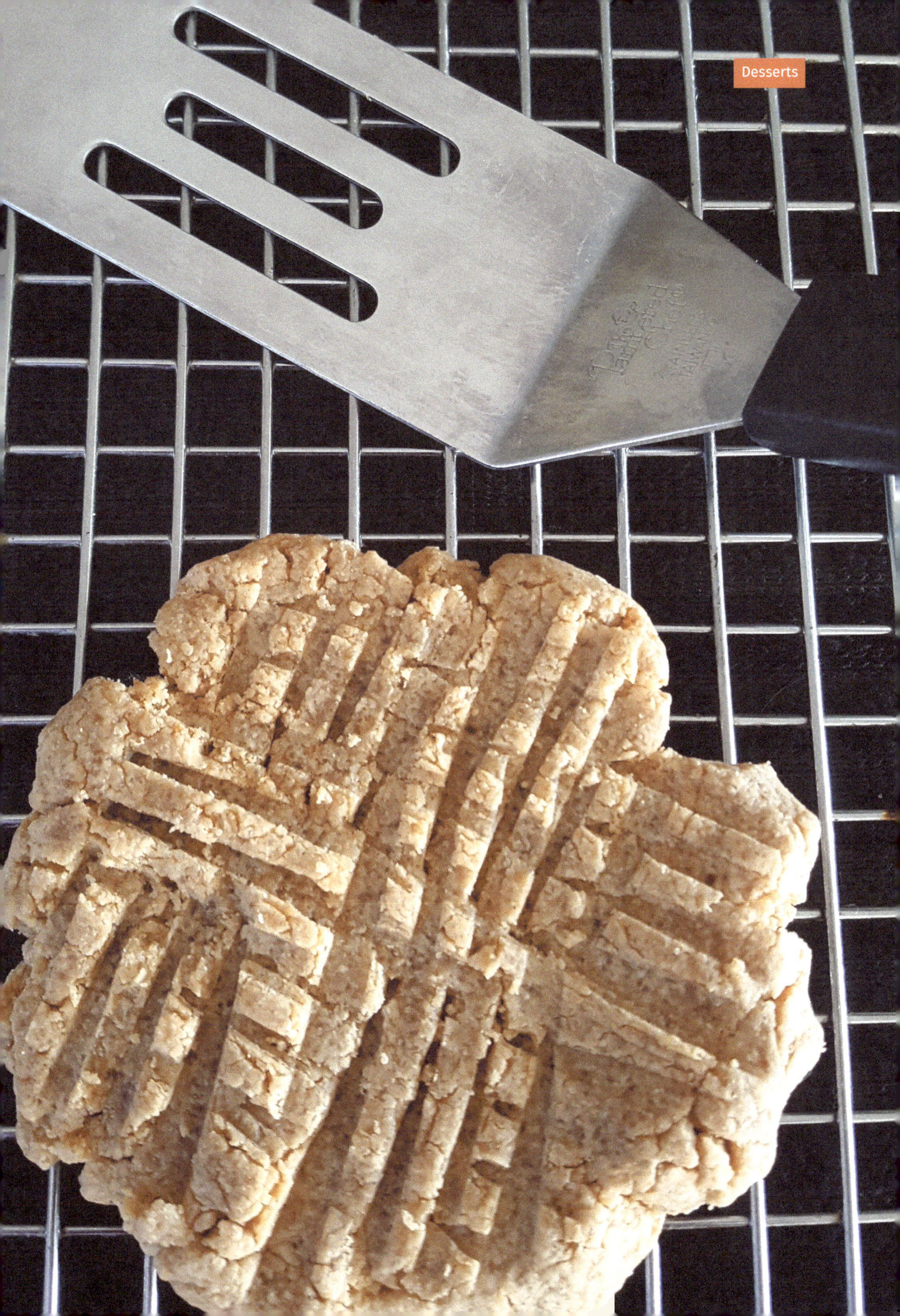

Desserts

COMFORT COOKING
for Bariatric Post-Ops and Everyone Else!

"TOOTSIE ROLL" PROTEIN CHEWS

I would have never believed it, but it is possible to make this from chocolate protein powder. I have always believed that necessity is the mother of invention, and this proves it. Enjoy!

INGREDIENTS

- 2 scoops chocolate protein powder (I use Kaizen whey isolate)
- ¼ c. peanut butter powder
- 1 T. Truvia Baking Blend
- 2 T. unsweetened cocoa powder
- 1 T. sugar-free caramel syrup
- 2 T. water

INSTRUCTIONS

1. In a small bowl, mix all ingredients until well combined.
2. Dough will be thick and malleable but very sticky. Lightly spray your hands to avoid major sticking. Knead the mass a few times in the bowl then roughly hand form a log and place it on a sheet of plastic wrap that has been sprayed with vegetable spray.
3. Fold over the plastic to completely wrap the log. Roll into a long tube and place into the fridge for one hour.
4. Cut into 18 bite-sized pieces. Store in the fridge.

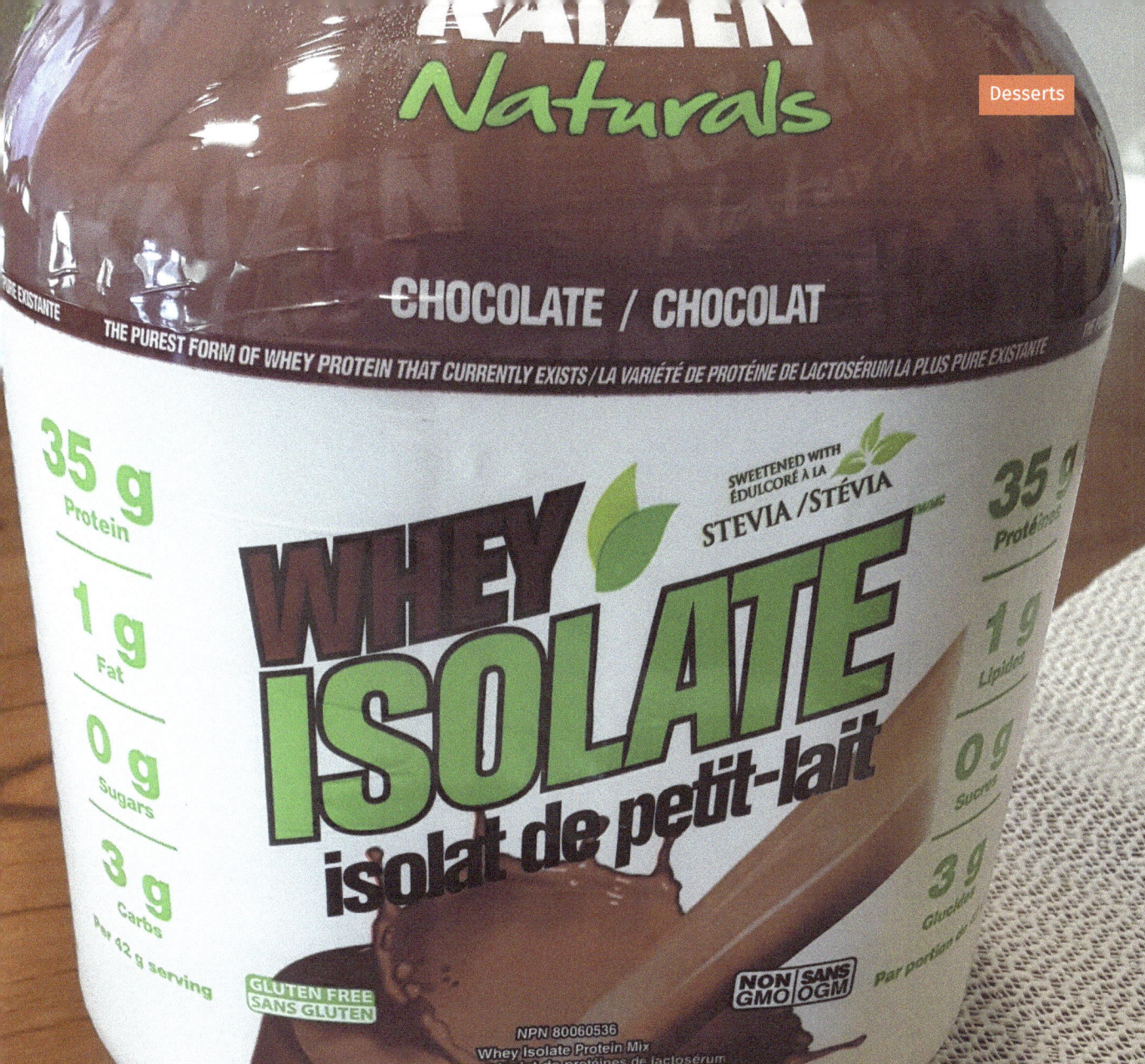

Desserts

COMFORT COOKING
for Bariatric Post-Ops and Everyone Else!

CRUNCHY PROTEIN CINNAMON CEREAL

Commercial cereals are a bariatric no-no because of the overload of carbs and added sugar. This recipe was developed out of necessity when I was desperate for a morning cinnamony crunch. It is like munching your morning protein shake! It even stays crunchy in milk!

INGREDIENTS

Makes one and one-quarter cups (serving size is one-half cup, approximately 30 grams of protein)

- 2 T. almond flour
- 2 scoops vanilla whey protein isolate powder
- (I use Kaizen whey isolate)
- 2 t. heaping, ground cinnamon
- 1 t. Truvia Brown Sugar Blend
- 2 t. Truvia Baking Blend
- 1 egg white
- Pinch of salt
- 1 t. sugar-free vanilla syrup
- 1 t. olive oil

INSTRUCTIONS

Pre-heat oven to 300°F.

1. Combine all ingredients into a medium-sized bowl. Use a fork to mix. Dough will be dry, so wet a finger or two (be careful not too much water) and knead in the bowl with one hand until ball forms. Dough should be slightly sticky.

2. Place the dough on a large sheet of parchment paper and flatten slightly with the palm of your hand. Cover with another sheet of parchment paper and roll out as thinly as possible. I use both a rolling pin and the flat side of a mallet to pound it out! (You need muscle here as dough is stiff!)

3. Remove the top parchment paper and transfer rolled out dough onto a cookie sheet. Bake for 15 minutes. Remove from oven and peel off the parchment paper. Using a large sharp knife, slice the entire dough into thin vertical strips then slice across horizontally to form small squares.

4. Coat the cookie sheet with vegetable spray and transfer the cereal squares back to the cookie sheet (no parchment paper). Lightly spray the top of the cereal with vegetable spray, then bake for an additional 10 minutes.

5. Remove from the oven and allow to cool on the sheet.

6. Place the cereal in a Ziploc bag to store. These are over-the-top crunchy and retain their crunch forever. I keep the bag unzipped. Eat as a crunchy protein snack, or with unsweetened almond milk in a bowl. If eating as a cereal in milk, same rules apply as for soup. Liquid first, chunks later! Enjoy!

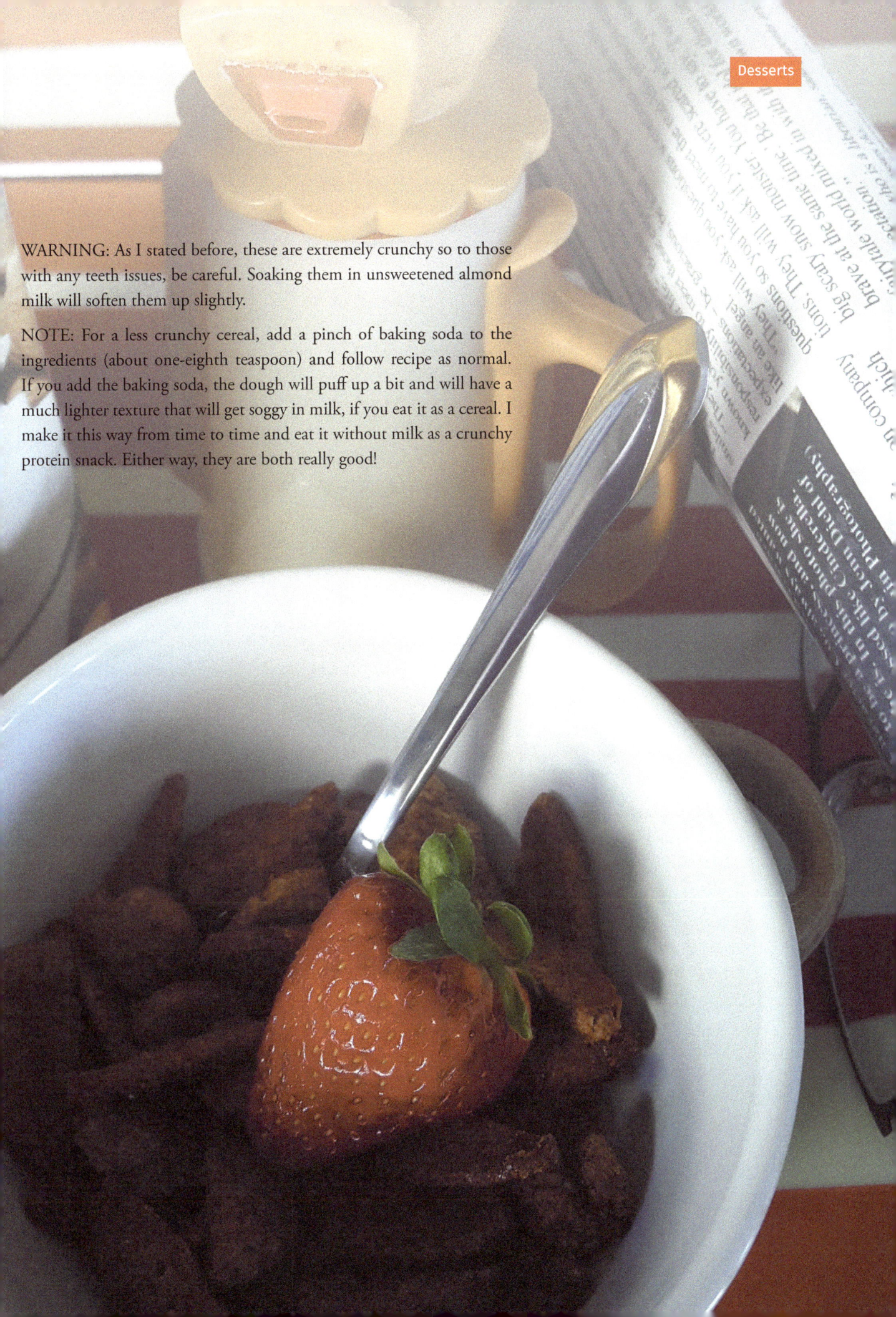

Desserts

WARNING: As I stated before, these are extremely crunchy so to those with any teeth issues, be careful. Soaking them in unsweetened almond milk will soften them up slightly.

NOTE: For a less crunchy cereal, add a pinch of baking soda to the ingredients (about one-eighth teaspoon) and follow recipe as normal. If you add the baking soda, the dough will puff up a bit and will have a much lighter texture that will get soggy in milk, if you eat it as a cereal. I make it this way from time to time and eat it without milk as a crunchy protein snack. Either way, they are both really good!

OH MY STRAWBERRY PIE (NO BAKE)

This is a makeover of a retro dessert from the '60s! Make this in the summer when fresh strawberries are at their finest. And, if you are invited to a BBQ party, offer to bring the dessert! It will be the hit of the party!

INGREDIENTS

1 10-oz. package sugar-free shortbread cookies (I use Peek Freans Lifestyle)

4 T. melted butter

¼ t. cinnamon

¼ c. plus 2 T. Truvia Baking Blend

2 ⅓ c. cold water

3 T. cornstarch

6 c. fresh strawberries, sliced

3 packages sugar-free strawberry Jell-O powder (I use 10-g. packages)

Sugar-free Cool Whip or your own no-sugar-added whipped cream

INSTRUCTIONS

1. Spray a 9-inch pie plate with cooking spray (I use a deep glass pie plate that measures 11 inches across, including the rim, with a 9-inch bottom).

2. In a food processor, pulse the cookies until they resemble fine crumbs. Add the butter, cinnamon, and one tablespoon Truvia. Pulse again, until the mixture resembles damp sand. Press into the bottom of the pie plate and up the sides, using a small measuring cup. Chill while filling is prepared.

3. Dissolve cold water, the remaining one-quarter cup plus one tablespoon Truvia and cornstarch in a medium-sized pot. Bring to a boil over medium heat, stirring frequently. Cook until clear, glossy and thickened, about two to three minutes.

4. Remove from heat and stir in the Jell-O powders, mixing until completely dissolved. Stir in two cups of strawberries and combine well. Give the remaining four cups of strawberries a few squirts of flavoured water enhancer (I use either strawberry or any berry flavour). This will infuse the strawberries with an extra level of flavour and aroma. It is optional; however, I recommend it.

5. Remove chilled crust and arrange the remaining four cups of strawberries on the crust. Carefully pour the hot mixture over the berries in the pie plate.

6. Chill for four hours or more. Cut into slices and serve with sugar-free whipped cream! Yummy!

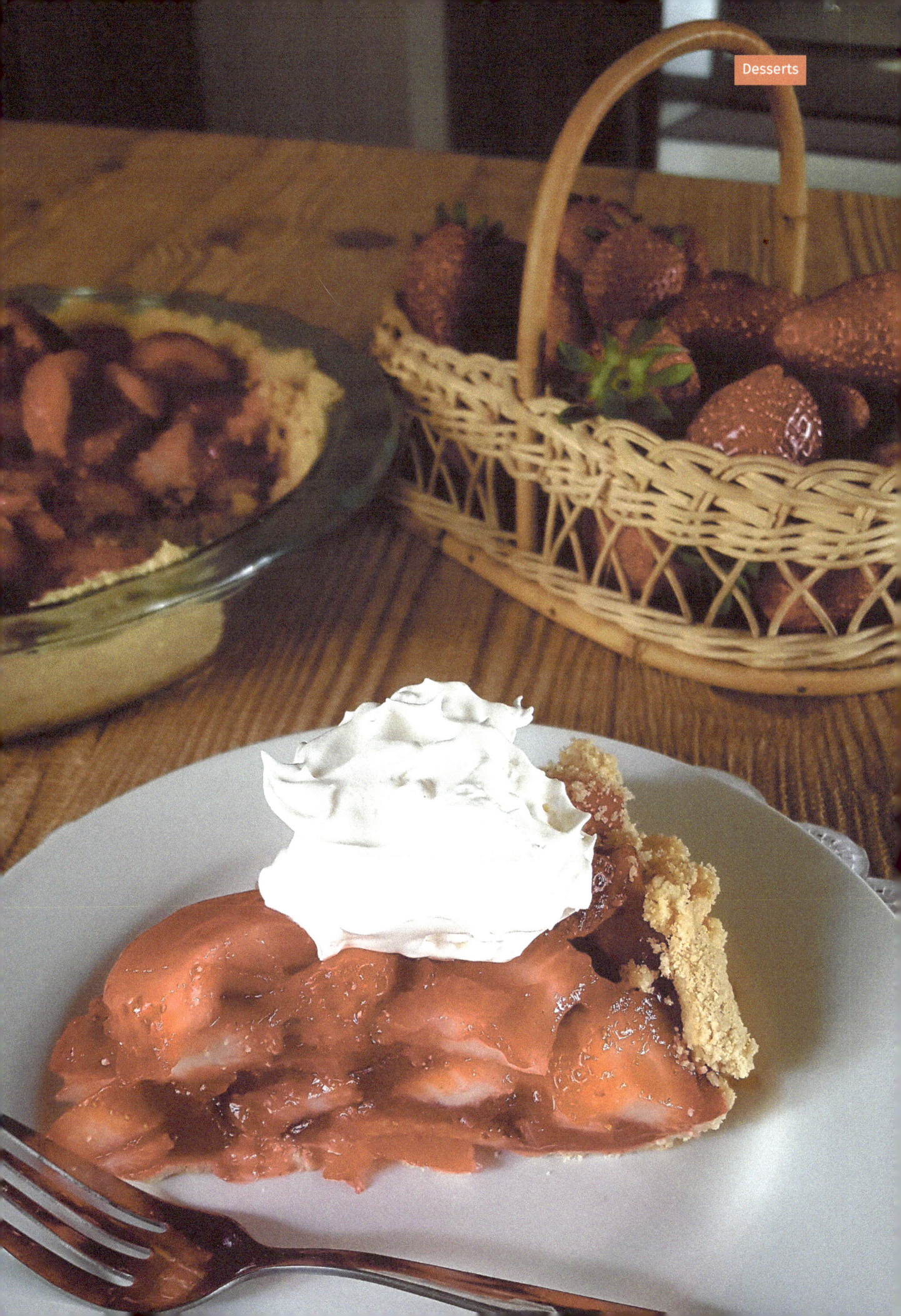

Desserts

RASPBERRY ITALIAN ICE

This is a lovely cool treat that can be served in an elegant glass, dessert bowl or made into popsicles. Whichever way you decide to serve it, enjoy!

INGREDIENTS

3–4 c. fresh berries (I like combining raspberries and blackberries)

Fresh lemon juice

Granular sweetener to taste

Sugar-free water enhancer (I use Nestle Nesfruta Raspberry)

INSTRUCTIONS

1. Place the fruit into your blender or food processor and puree the fruit until smooth. Transfer to a 9 × 9 metal cake pan, add juice of half a lemon and sweeten to taste. I also give a squirt of a water enhancer in a berry flavour. Mix everything well.

2. Place the pan into the freezer and, every 15 minutes or so, remove from the freezer and with a fork, blend the ice crystals as they form, scraping the fruit upward, like raking grass. Do this until the entire pan is scraped up and fruit is slushy. It is now ready to serve! If you leave it longer in the freezer, the mixture will freeze solid. When this happens, place the pan on your counter and let it thaw slightly until you are able to scrape the crystals.

NOTE: If you want to make popsicles, just pour the prepared fruit puree into moulds, and freeze as you normally would.

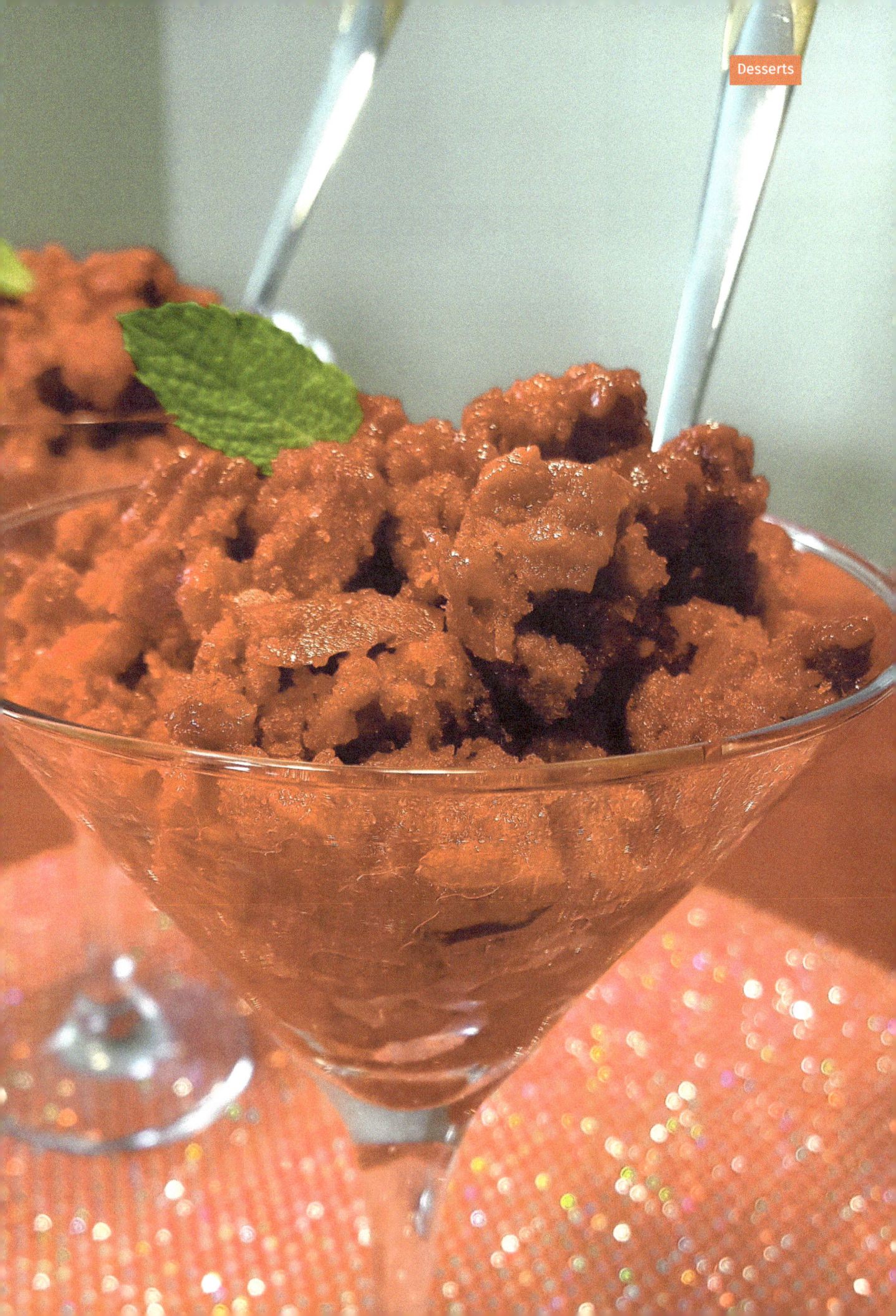

Desserts

REFERENCES

O'Connor, Anahad. "How the Sugar Industry Shifted Blame to Fat." *New York Times*, September 12, 2016.

Davis, William M.D. *Wheat Belly*. New York (NY): RODALE; 2011. p 125.

MY BFF

I AM FORTUNATE TO HAVE BEEN HANDED DOWN A VERY OLD '70S CONTRAPTION CALLED A "MOULI." I grew up with this thing and I have fond memories of my mom using it. It is one of the most primitive graters that I have ever seen, and to this day, it does a better job than any other gadget out there. You crank the handle, which turns the blade that grates whatever you've put inside. It IS my BFF and I would be lost without it. My Mouli bears the scars of time and I will treasure it till death do us part. I mostly use it to grate my cauliflower and cheese. Of course, your food processor does the same job as my beloved Mouli, but I will say without a doubt, it is nowhere near as much fun!

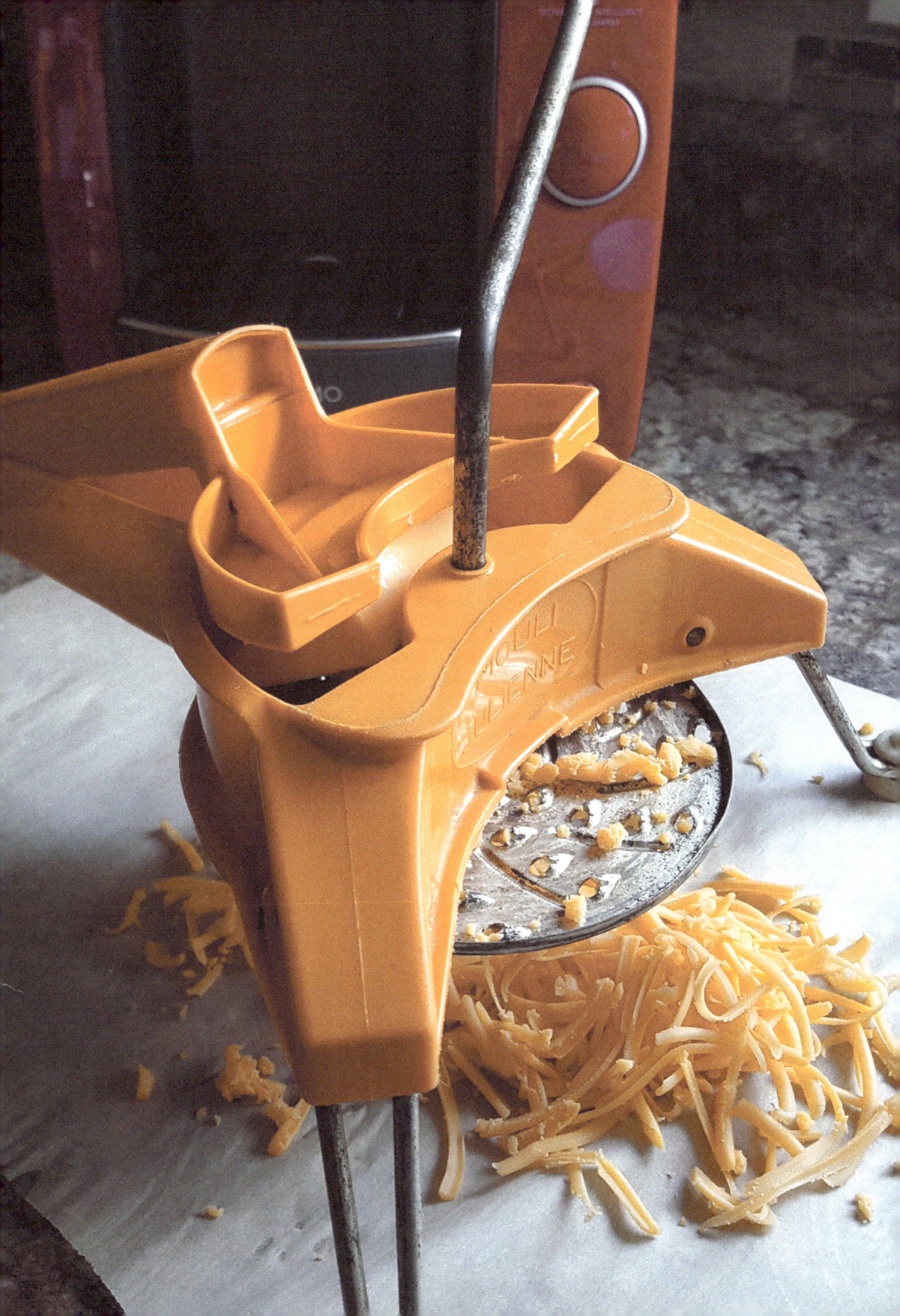

ABOUT THE AUTHOR

BORN IN WINNIPEG, CANADA, LISA SHARON BELKIN GREW UP IN AN ARTISTIC HOUSEHOLD. BOTH OF her parents were members of the Winnipeg Symphony Orchestra, and the family environment was heavily focused on music and the visual arts. Ms. Belkin is a teacher by profession and an accomplished sculptor, painter, and author. Three years after her bariatric surgery, she found herself making bad choices and the foods that grew her to almost 400 pounds began creeping back into her life. She belongs to several bariatric support groups and is closely connected to many post-ops who are struggling with their food choices and are facing weight regain. With *Comfort Cooking for Bariatric Post-Ops and Everyone Else!*, Lisa's goal is two-fold: to help others who are struggling to be successful after bariatric surgery and to increase awareness that surgery is not an easy way out. Her last book, *The Cosmetics Cookbook* (available on Amazon), was on Canadian bookstore McNally Robinson's bestsellers list in 1998. Numerous recipes and beauty tips from the book were featured in the popular American magazine *Woman's World* and several Canadian publications. Ms. Belkin graduated from the University of Manitoba with degrees in both Education and Counselling. She currently resides in Saskatoon, Canada, with her partner, Randy, and their two cats, Ozzie and Tigger.

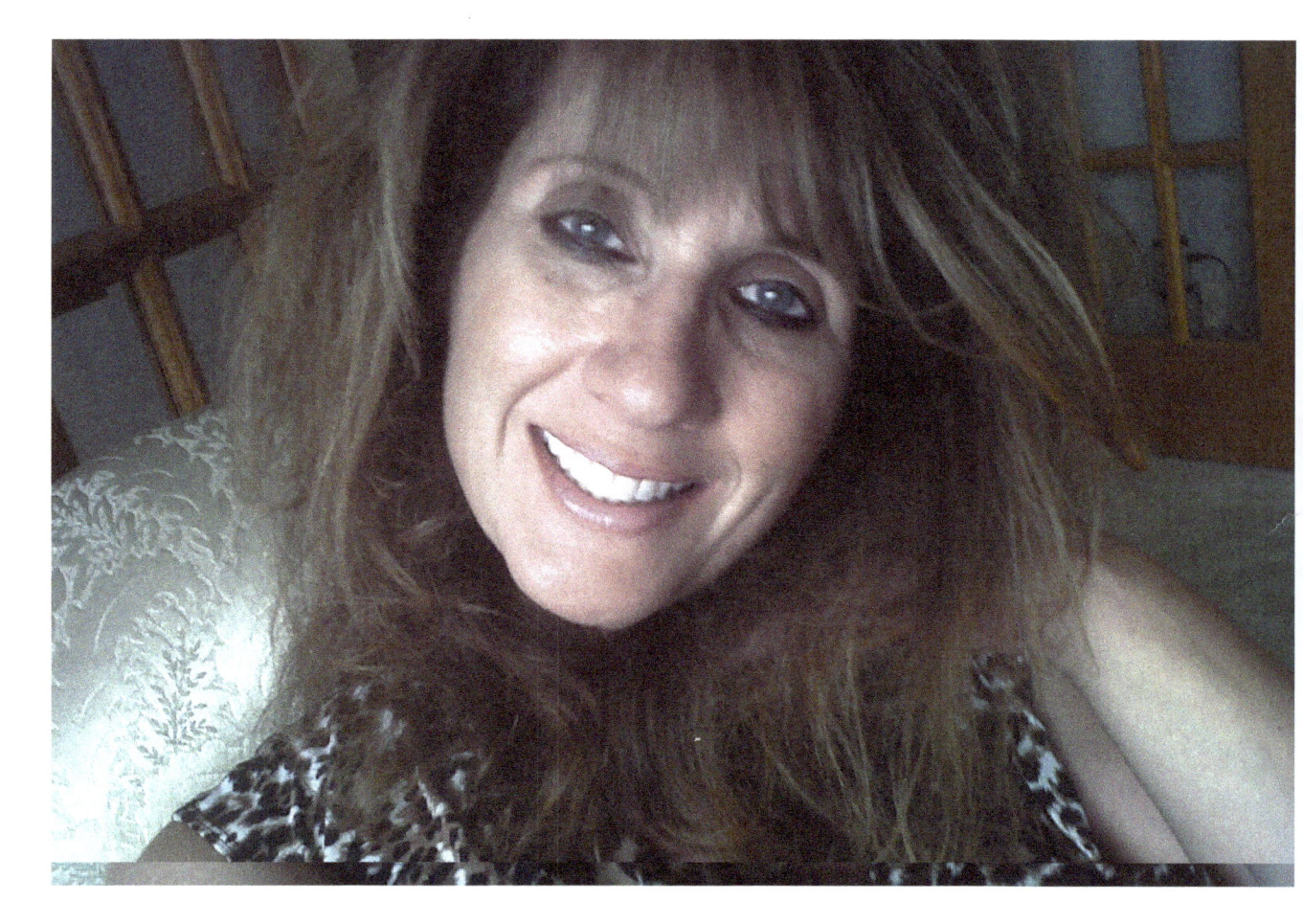